Leg Ulcers:

Nursing Management

A Research-based Guide

Leg Ulcers:
Nursing Management

A Research-based Guide

EDITED BY

Nicky Cullum

PhD, RGN
Lecturer in Nursing, University of Liverpool

and

Brenda Roe

PhD, RGN
Senior Research Fellow, Health Services Research Unit, University of Oxford

Produced with an educational grant
from Smith & Nephew Medical Limited

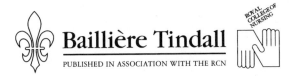

Baillière Tindall
PUBLISHED IN ASSOCIATION WITH THE RCN

Baillière Tindall   24–28 Oval Road
London NW1 7DX

The Curtis Center
Independence Square West
Philadelphia, PA 19106-3399, USA

Harcourt Brace & Company
55 Horner Avenue
Toronto, Ontario M8Z 4X6, Canada

Harcourt Brace & Company, Australia
30–52 Smidmore Street
Marrickville
NSW 2204, Australia

Harcourt Brace & Company, Japan
Ichibancho Central Building
22-1 Ichibancho
Chiyoda-ku, Tokyo 102, Japan

First printed 1995 by Scutari Press

A catalogue record for this book is available from the British Library

ISBN 1-871364-97-3

Printed and bound in Great Britain by WBC Book Manufacturers Ltd,
Bridgend, Mid Glamorgan

Contributors

Janice Cameron, RGN ONC FETC, Senior Nurse, Dermatology Unit, Slade Hospital, Oxford

Nicky Cullum, PhD RGN, Lecturer in Nursing, University of Liverpool

Jackie Dale, MSc RGN RCNT DipN(Lond), Area Nursing Officer, Lothian Health Board

Astrid Fletcher, PhD, Senior Lecturer in Epidemiology, London School of Hygiene and Tropical Medicine

Barbara Gibson, SRN SCM, Leg Ulcer Specialist, Falkirk and District Royal Infirmary

Claire Louise Hamer, BSc(Hons) RGN, Research Assistant, Institute of Human Ageing, Liverpool

Julia V Keachie, SRN, Community Staff Nurse, Arran War Memorial Hospital, Lamlash, Isle of Arran

Christine J Moffatt, RGN NDN, Director, Riverside Venous Ulcer Service, London

Andrea Nelson, BSc(Hons) RGN, Research Associate, Lothian and Forth Valley Leg Ulcer Study Group

Stephen Thomas, BPharm PhD MRPharmS, Director, Surgical Materials Testing Laboratory, Bridgend General Hospital

Brenda Roe, PhD RGN, Senior Research Fellow, Health Services Research Unit, University of Oxford

Contents

Preface ix

Foreword xi

List of Colour Plates xii

1 The Anatomy and Physiology of the Circulation of the Leg 1
   Jackie Dale

2 The Aetiology of Leg Ulceration 9
   Jackie Dale

3 The Epidemiology of Leg Ulcers 17
   Astrid Fletcher

4 The Nursing Assessment of Patients with Leg Ulcers 27
   Barbara Gibson

5 Topical Applications in Leg Ulcer Management 35
   Nicky Cullum

6 Bandages Used in Leg Ulcer Management 63
   Stephen Thomas

7 The Art and Science of Bandaging 75
   Andrea Nelson

8 Prevention of Re-ulceration 89
   Julia Keachie

9 Contact Sensitivity and Eczema in Leg Ulcer Patients 101
   Janice Cameron

10 The Management of Leg Ulcers: Current Nursing Practice 113
   Brenda Roe and Nicky Cullum

11 Patients' Perceptions of Chronic Leg Ulceration 125
   Brenda Roe, Nicky Cullum and Claire Hamer

12   The Organisation and Delivery of Leg Ulcer Care.   135
        Christine Moffatt

13   Leg Ulcer Research and Practice: The Way Forward 149
        Nicky Cullum and Brenda Roe
        Index   155

Preface

Leg ulcers have been recognised by the Department of Health, health professionals and research scientists as a priority area for clinical practice and research. It has been roughly estimated that 1 per cent of the adult population in the UK is affected by leg ulceration at some time. This not only has sizeable implications for treatment costs and professionals' time but also personal costs for the sufferers. Community nurses, as key members of the primary health care team, are the main sources of care, with more than 84 per cent of district nurses' time spent in the treatment of leg ulcers. It is imperative that all nursing care is based on sound research evidence. This book provides a comprehensive review of the research on the nursing management of leg ulcers. The participating authors are acknowledged experts in this field, having contributed notable research and developments in clinical practice. Each chapter stands alone and covers an indepth aspect of leg ulcers and their management, and as such forms a basis for the planning and provision of nursing care for patients with this chronic condition.

Jackie Dale has presented two chapters (chapters 1 and 2) on the anatomy and physiology of leg circulation, and the pathology of leg ulceration. These chapters present an overview of the normal structure and function of lower limb circulation along with a description of the pathological processes which may result in the formation of the various types of leg ulcer. Astrid Fletcher (chapter 3) reviews what is known of the epidemiology of venous disease and leg ulceration. Barbara Gibson (chapter 4) presents a detailed guide to the nursing assessment of a patient presenting with leg ulceration. Such an expert assessment is essential to determine the subsequent care. Nicky Cullum (chapter 5) reviews the research which under-pins the use of topical agents, including wound dressings, in leg ulcer management. Steve Thomas (chapter 6) presents the theory of compression bandaging, a detailed description of bandage typology and a critical review of relevant clinical trials. Andrea Nelson (chapter 7) takes this subject further when she applies this theory to bandaging practice, describing the art of bandage application and the variables which determine sub-bandage pressure. Julia Keachie (née Cornwall) (chapter 8) describes strategies aimed at preventing re-ulceration, including the issue of compression hosiery. Janice Cameron (chapter 9) describes the problem of allergic reactions such as contact sensitivity and eczema to treatment in leg ulcer patients, and how they may be alleviated. Brenda Roe and Nicky Cullum (chapter 10) describe key studies which have investigated the current nursing management of patients with leg ulcers in the community. Brenda Roe, Nicky Cullum and Claire Hamer (chapter 11) describe a unique exploration of patients' knowledge and experience of having leg ulceration and its impact on their well-being and lifestyle.

Christine Moffatt (chapter 12) describes the varying approaches to the organization and delivery of nursing care to leg ulcer patients, with emphasis on the implementation of community clinics. Finally, Nicky Cullum and Brenda Roe (chapter 13) make suggestions for the way forward in leg ulcer research, and discuss the need for the identification of appropriate research questions and the use of sound research designs. Although each chapter stands alone as a summary of the knowledge in a particular area, the sum of the whole represents a vital guide to the effective and efficient nursing management of patients with leg ulcers.

Nicky Cullum and Brenda Roe

Foreword

Everyone managing leg ulcers will welcome a book which so carefully reviews the literature and indicates so clearly which data so far published is reliable and which is not. It exposes our ignorance and indicates exactly where more studies are needed. The authors have already gained a reputation for the analysis of the controlled trials in this field. It is an analysis which is timely and I welcome the fact that it has been performed by the nursing profession. Management at the interface with the patient is a nursing role. This book emphasises that where the diagnosis is difficult or the management invasive, the medical profession should be called in at an early stage. Conversely, the medical profession should be able to trust the nurse to provide good management based on scientific evidence rather than on whim. If every nurse and every doctor were to review this book as carefully as I have done before writing the foreword, their management would at least be based on the best evidence available and, as such, this would be a big leap forward.

Terence J Ryan
Clinical Professor of Dermatology

List of Colour Plates

Plate 1: Venous staining, varicose veins and ankle flare

Plate 2: Ischaemic leg with shiny, hairless skin

Plate 3: Dorsalis pedis pulse

Plate 4: Posterior tibial pulse

Plate 5: Doppler ultrasound

Plate 6: Venous ulcer

Plate 7: Arterial ulcer

Plate 8: Diabetic foot with ulcerated toe

Plate 9: Rheumatoid ulcer

Plate 10: Malignant ulcer

Plate 11: Skin damage on foot due to pressure

Plates 12, 13, 14: Bandaging the foot

Plates 15, 16: Spiral bandaging of the leg

Plate 17: Figure of eight bandaging

Plate 18: Measuring bandage overlap

Plate 19: Padding the gaiter

Plate 20: Foam protecting the foot

Plate 21: Skin damage at the edge of a dressing

Plate 22: A leg ulcer surrounded by stasis eczema

Plate 23: Test strips applied to a patient's back

Plate 24: A positive patch test

1

The Anatomy and Physiology
of the Circulation of the Leg

A sound knowledge of the anatomy of the vascular system of the leg is essential for the understanding of how leg ulcers are formed and how they can be treated; most leg ulcers are a result of vascular disease. Disease affecting the arteries, veins or lymphatics may contribute; however, it is venous disease which is most commonly associated with leg ulceration (Callam et al, 1987).

THE VASCULAR SYSTEM OF THE LEG

There are four main types of vessels forming the vascular system of the leg: arteries, veins, capillaries and lymphatics. The arteries carry oxygenated blood from the heart to the capillary bed, where oxygen and nutrients are exchanged for carbon dioxide and waste products from the tissues. Deoxygenated blood is returned to the heart in the veins. The lymphatic network returns interstitial fluid and other plasma constituents such as protein molecules, back into the systemic circulation.

Arteries

An adult has approximately 5 l of blood, about 15 per cent of which is contained in the arteries (Guyton, 1991). Blood flow in the arteries is rapid, but varies in different parts of the body and according to the level of muscular activity. Arteries have strong muscular walls which can relax or constrict in response to the autonomic nervous system and thus regulate blood flow. Large arteries divide and subdivide into smaller vessels, known as arterioles, as they extend into the tissues. Diseased arterioles may cause some types of leg ulcers.

Capillaries

The capillaries are the smallest vessels and body function is entirely dependent on them. Oxygen, nutrients and waste products are exchanged between the tissues and the blood through their thin walls. The sole function of the heart and larger blood vessels is to maintain an adequate blood flow through the capillaries.

The amount of blood held in the capillary bed (about 5 per cent of total blood volume) plays an important part in the control of body temperature and blood pressure. Blood moves slowly through the capillaries at a pressure of about 35 mmHg. The capillary diameter, and thus the rate of flow, is controlled by the autonomic nervous system.

Veins and Venules

Veins and venules have thinner, less muscular walls than arteries and can dilate to accommodate up to about 80 per cent of the total blood volume if necessary. Venous blood pressure is affected by gravity and changes in the body position. When a person is standing upright the pressure in the deep leg veins is about 90 mmHg, depending on the length of the column of blood between the foot and the heart (ie. the height of the individual). When recumbent, the pressure is only about 10 mmHg (see figure 1.1).

An important feature of the leg veins is the presence of one-way valves. These are semi-lunar folds of the smooth endothelium, with which all blood vessels are lined. These folds project into the lumen of the vessel in the form of paired cusps. The wall of the vein where the cusps are attached forms a slight bulge, called the venous sinus, which can be seen in venograms (see figure 1.2).

Obstruction or back-pressure on the veins causes a rise in pressure in the capillaries which results in increased filtration of protein-containing fluid into the surrounding tissue spaces.

Lymphatics

The lymph vessels are thin-walled, rather like the capillaries but they arise blindly in the tissues and form a network, with individual vessels merging to become bigger as they progress. Their paths usually lie close to the blood vessels. Lymph vessels have a knotty appearance due to the presence of valves similar to those in the veins.

Lymph is a protein-rich fluid resembling blood plasma and, like venous blood, is propelled by muscle movement. The function of the lymphatics is to drain excess tissue fluid back into the blood vessels but their capacity is limited and oedema is formed when the volume of tissue fluid is too great. Gross oedema (lymphoedema) occurs if the lymphatics have been blocked by the spread of carcinoma, damaged by infection or have been surgically removed.

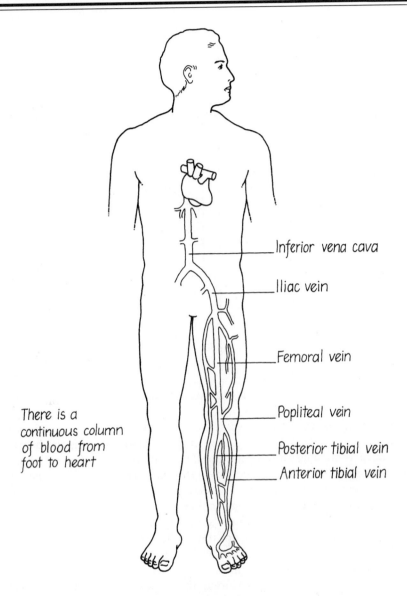

There is a
continuous column
of blood from
foot to heart

Inferior vena cava

Iliac vein

Femoral vein

Popliteal vein

Posterior tibial vein

Anterior tibial vein

Fig 1.1 The deep veins

The Venous Circulation and the Calf Muscle Pump

The mechanism by which blood returning from the legs is propelled against the force of gravity is known as *the calf muscle pump*. The pump has four components which work together to propel the blood back to the heart. These are: the deep veins, the superficial veins, the valves and the calf muscle inside its tough inelastic sheath (the fascia).

The deep and superficial venous systems are connected at various points by

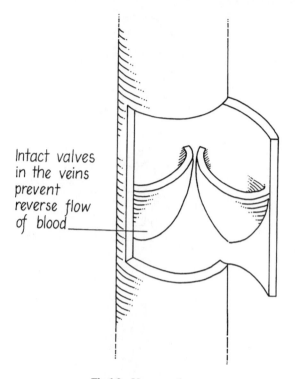

Intact valves
in the veins
prevent
reverse flow
of blood

Fig 1.2   Venous valves

communicating veins. All these vessels contain one-way valves which seal off the vein if there is any back-flow, thus directing the blood towards the heart.

The **deep veins**, consisting of the popliteal and femoral veins, carry most of the blood returning from the leg and can withstand high pressures as they are thick-walled, surrounded by muscle and lie deep within the fascia.

The **superficial veins** are the long saphenous vein, extending up the medial side of the leg from foot to groin, and the short saphenous vein running up the back of the calf from foot to knee. They are thin-walled, are not supported by muscle, lie outside the fascia and cannot withstand high pressures.

The **communicating veins** of the lower leg (sometimes called the 'perforators' because they pass through, or perforate, the muscle fascia) join the superficial and deep veins and are relatively large with thicker walls.

The **blood is propelled back to the heart by the changes in shape of calf muscles as the leg moves**. During dorsiflexion, the calf muscle contracts, becoming shorter and thicker. The forces are directed inwards because the muscle is enclosed in the unyielding fascia. The muscle compresses the deep vein and increases the pressure within it. This closes the one-way valves and forces venous blood up towards the heart, emptying the deep veins. Backflow of blood into the superficial veins is prevented by the presence of valves in the perforators, *provided that those valves are undamaged and competent*. During plantarflexion, the muscle relaxes and the veins refill, so that the cycle can begin again (see figure 1.3).

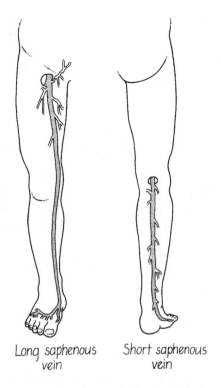

Long saphenous
vein

Short saphenous
vein

Fig 1.3 The main superficial veins of the leg

This description of the way in which the leg muscles, veins and valves act together to form a pump is necessarily over-simplified. In fact several muscle pumps have been described in the lower limb. Gardner and Fox (1985) used video phlebography to identify a separate mechanism triggered by the intermittent stretching of the plantar veins during foot movement. They have called this the foot pump and have shown that it is independent of calf muscle movement by demonstrating it in paralysed limbs.

In practical terms, this means that walking is the most effective way to activate the calf and foot pumps, and it follows that patients with venous problems should be encouraged to walk as much as possible (see figure 1.4).

The efficiency of the pumps depends on competent valves preventing the blood from flowing back down the leg (venous reflux). The valves may be damaged by trauma, or more usually, by an episode of deep venous thrombosis (DVT). Although the vein may recanalise and allow the passage of blood once more, the valves may be completely destroyed and at best will never fully recover. The valves in the perforators are the most important. While these are still intact, ulcer formation is unlikely (see figure 1.5).

The anatomy of the leg veins is not the same on both sides of the body. It is suggested that deep venous thrombosis is much more frequent in the left leg than the right because the left common iliac vein is subject to pressure as it passes

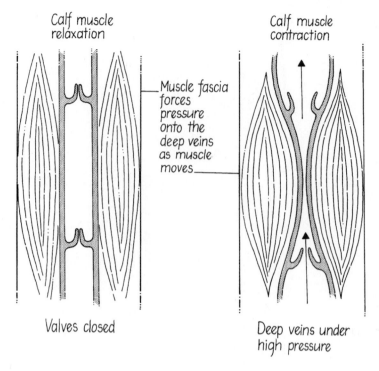

Calf muscle
relaxation

Calf muscle
contraction

Muscle fascia
forces
pressure
onto the
deep veins
as muscle
moves

Valves closed

Deep veins under
high pressure

Fig 1.4 The calf muscles provide the power that propels blood back to the heart

between the body of the fifth lumbar vertebra and the right common iliac artery at the junction with the vena cava. This may be the reason why leg ulcers occur more frequently on the left leg than on the right (Negus and Walters, 1991).

SUMMARY

- Most leg ulcers are caused by vascular disease.
- Blood pressure is highest in the arteries and lowest in the capillaries and superficial veins. Oedema is a consequence of back-pressure from the veins to the capillaries.
- All veins contain one-way valves which prevent venous reflux when intact.
- The calf muscle pump is the mechanism which clears venous blood from the legs and maintains the blood pressures in the deep and superficial veins at the correct levels.
- The calf muscle pump is powered by leg movements.
- The efficiency of the calf muscle pump depends on the patency of the venous valves.
- Venous valves can be damaged, irreparably, by deep venous thrombosis.

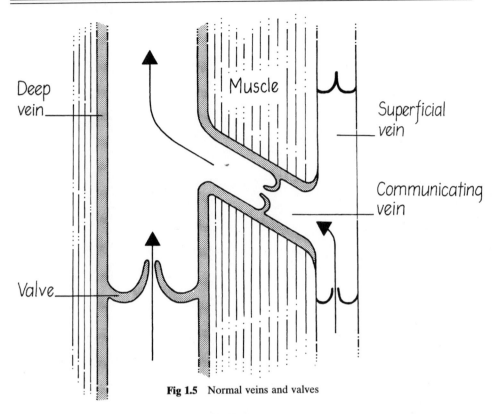

Fig 1.5   Normal veins and valves

References

Callam M J, Harper D R, Dale J J and Ruckley C V (1987) Chronic ulcer of the leg: clinical
history. *British Medical Journal*, **290**: 1855–1856.
Gardner A M N and Fox R H (1985) The return of blood to the heart against gravity. In:
Phlebology '85, eds Negus D and Jantet G. London: Libbey.
Guyton A C (1991) *Human Physiology and the Mechanisms of Disease*, pp. 111–112, 5th
edn. Philadelphia: W B Saunders.
Negus D and Walters H (1991) *Leg Ulcers: A Practical Approach to Management*. Oxford:
Butterworth-Heinemann.

Bibliography

Hamilton W J (1982) *Textbook of Human Anatomy*. London: Macmillan.
Williams P L, Warwick R, Dyson M and Bannister L H (1989) *Gray's Anatomy*. Edinburgh:
Churchill Livingstone.

2

The Aetiology of Leg

Ulceration

WHAT IS A LEG ULCER?

Giving something a name implies that we know enough about it to classify it; however, when first seeing a patient with a leg ulcer it is wise to keep an open mind as to the cause. Leg ulcers have many causes and have been known under a variety of names historically; however, some of these names are misleading. For practical purposes we need a neutral term and non-judgemental general definition. The following definition, which has been used in an epidemiological study (Dale et al, 1983) is useful because it is simple and makes no assumption as to the cause of ulceration:

"A leg ulcer is a loss of skin below the knee on the leg or foot which takes more than 6 weeks to heal."

This should be the starting point from which to consider all leg ulcers.

Six hundred patients examined during a large survey in Scotland were found to have the conditions shown in table 2.1 associated with leg ulceration. The fact that the right hand column totals more than 100 per cent indicates that some patients had ulcers of mixed aetiology, where more than one factor was present.

Table 2.1 Factors associated with leg ulceration

Venous disease	70%
Arterial disease	22%
Rheumatoid arthritis	8.5%
Diabetes	5.5%
Burns	2.5%
Infections	1%
Blood disease	1%
Lymphoedema	0.5%
Malignant disease	rare

From Callam et al (1985).

More recently, while examining patients for inclusion in a randomised, controlled clinical trial we have been able to quantify the groups more accurately (unpublished data). The largest group comprises patients with purely venous ulcers (59 per cent); these can be treated conservatively by nurses with minimal medical intervention, provided that the diagnosis is in no doubt. The next important group, which includes patients with peripheral vascular disease and diabetes as underlying causes, comprises patients with arterial ulcers. These constitute about 21 per cent of ulcers. The last major group consists of patients with 'mixed' ulcers (20 per cent), where venous, arterial, rheumatoid arthritis and other diseases play a part. It is necessary to assess the relative importance of each contributing factor in patients with ulcers of mixed aetiology, and this is a medical responsibility.

Venous Ulcers

Venous disease is so common amongst the general population, that although it does not inevitably lead to ulceration, it is not surprising that venous ulcers are the most frequently seen. There are a few ulcers which result from primary superficial varicose veins, and which could legitimately be called 'varicose'. When varicose ulcers occur they heal quickly with simple conservative treatment and may clear up spontaneously if the small vein involved becomes thrombosed in the natural course of events. The vast majority of venous ulcers, however, are secondary to long-established disease of the deep veins (Burnand and Browse, 1982).

Normally the resting pressure in the veins of the foot in the erect posture is about 80–90 mmHg, falling to about 25 mmHg after the activation of the calf muscle pump by exercise of the leg muscles. If, however, damaged or incompetent valves in the perforating veins allow back flow of blood (at relatively high pressure) into the thin-walled superficial veins, then the superficial veins become stretched and dilated (see figure 2.1). This, in itself, exacerbates the venous insufficiency, since the distance between the flaps of any remaining competent valves is increased, and a whole series of valves will fail to close properly. As a result there is a back-flow of blood and an increased hydrostatic pressure in the superficial veins, which is transmitted to the capillaries. The single-celled capillary walls become stretched, leading to abnormal leakage of fluids into the tissues and skin.

The effects of increased capillary permeability are (see figure 2.2):

- Oedema caused by the loss of water and plasma proteins to the tissues.
- Leakage of red blood cells which release haemoglobin into the tissues as they disintegrate.
- Irritation of the skin and eczema caused by the breakdown products of haemoglobin.
- Skin staining from the breakdown of haemoglobin.

Fibrinogen from the leaked plasma is also deposited in the tissues as insoluble fibrin complexes which surround the capillaries and may prevent the exchange of oxygen and nutrients so causing tissue death. These complexes are sometimes described as 'fibrin cuffs' (Burnand et al, 1982). The result of this process, affecting the skin and the veins supplying the skin, is known as lipodermatosclerosis. If advanced lipodermatosclerosis is present, the leg feels hard and woody, or 'indurated' beneath the skin, where the fibrin has been deposited.

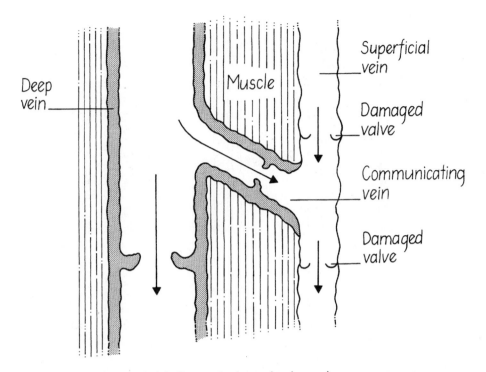

Fig 2.1 Damaged valves and varicose veins

The fibrin cuff hypothesis explains many of the observable skin and tissue changes associated with venous ulcers, but some researchers now suggest that capillary blocking by trapped white blood cells may also be involved in skin breakdown (Coleridge-Smith et al, 1988).

Ischaemic Ulcers

Arterial or ischaemic ulcers are caused by a blockage of one of the smaller arteries causing a loss of blood flow to the area of skin normally supplied by that artery. The skin, depleted of oxygen and nutrients becomes ischaemic and will eventually break down. If the onset of ischaemia is sudden, the blockage may be due to an embolism. Peripheral arterial disease, where the deposition of fatty substances (atheromatous plaques) in the arterial wall causes narrowing of the arterioles and eventual blockage of the vessel, is a more gradual process. Smoking exacerbates the condition. The prevalence of peripheral arterial disease increases with age, therefore it must be remembered that older patients with predominantly venous ulcers may also have some arterial insufficiency.

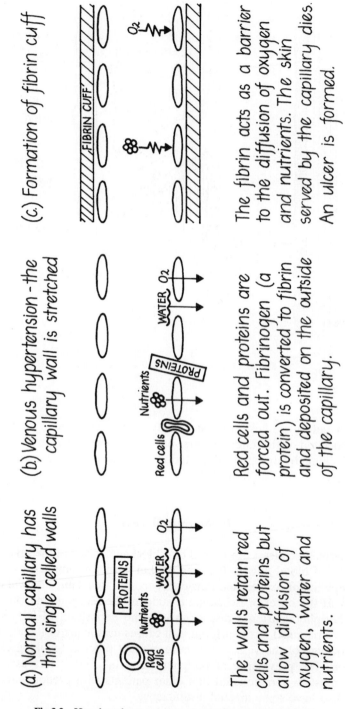

(a) Normal capillary has thin single celled walls

The walls retain red cells and proteins but allow diffusion of oxygen, water and nutrients.

(b) Venous hypertension - the capillary wall is stretched

Red cells and proteins are forced out. Fibrinogen (a protein) is converted to fibrin and deposited on the outside of the capillary.

(c) Formation of fibrin cuff

The fibrin acts as a barrier to the diffusion of oxygen and nutrients. The skin served by the capillary dies. An ulcer is formed.

Fig 2.2   How leg ulcers are formed—the fibrin cuff hypothesis

Diabetic Ulcers

Diabetic ulcers have many features in common with arterial ulcers. The complications of diabetes often include local arterial constriction or occlusion. In addition, diabetic neuropathy may cause anaesthetised, insensitive skin, in which injury may go unnoticed. Both arterial disease and neuropathy contribute to and cause ulceration.

Rheumatoid Arthritis

The reason why patients with rheumatoid arthritis develop leg ulcers is not completely understood, but it is thought to be a combination of local vasculitis, poor venous return due to immobility of the ankle joint and the debilitating effect of prolonged steroid therapy on the skin. The lack of understanding of the underlying pathology makes rheumatoid ulcers extremely difficult to treat.

Traumatic Ulcers

Some leg ulcers start with trauma in the gaiter area, often due to a knock from a supermarket trolley. The fact that such ulcers persist is probably due to the existence of underlying venous insufficiency or arterial disease. Burns caused by sitting too close to an open fire, sometimes known as 'grannie's tartan', may occasionally be a contributing cause amongst elderly women. Young men who fracture their legs in sporting or industrial accidents occasionally suffer from severe leg ulcers for the rest of their lives, especially if the veins were damaged and the injury was complicated by deep venous thrombosis.

Haemolytic Ulcers

Sickle cell anaemia, which distorts the shape and increases the fragility of red blood cells, is sometimes a cause of leg ulceration amongst people of Afro-caribbean descent.

Malignant Ulcers

Although malignant ulcers are rare, an existing ulcer may become malignant or an existing skin tumour may become ulcerated. Callam et al (1985) found none in their survey, but sufficient numbers have been identified and confirmed by biopsy for the possibility of malignancy to be considered where the ulcer is of unusual appearance or where it fails to heal in spite of every effort.

SUMMARY

- The four factors most often associated with leg ulceration are venous disease, arterial disease, diabetes mellitus and rheumatoid arthritis.
- Venous ulcers occur if incompetent valves in the perforating veins permit reflux of blood from the deep to the superficial veins and cause an increase in intra-capillary pressure. This is known as chronic venous insufficiency.
- Embolism or arteriosclerosis may block peripheral arteries or arterioles and cause ischaemic ulcers (see figure 2.3).
- Many ulcers have several contributing factors, and it is necessary to identify and assess each one.

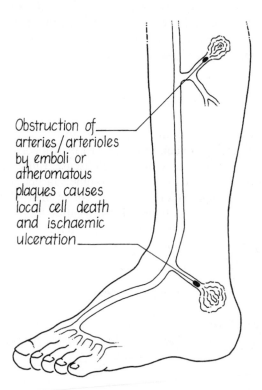

Obstruction of arteries/arterioles by emboli or atheromatous plaques causes local cell death and ischaemic ulceration

Fig 2.3   Ulcers may be caused by arterial obstruction, due to emboli or atheromatous plaques

References

Burnand K G, Whimster I, Naidoo A and Browse N L (1982) Pericapillary fibrin in the ulcer-bearing skin of the leg: the cause of lipodermatosclerosis and venous ulceration. *British Medical Journal*, **285**: 1071–1072.

Burnand K G and Browse N L (1982) The post-phlebitic limb and venous ulceration. *Recent Advances in Surgery 11*. London: Churchill Livingstone.

Callam M J, Ruckley C V, Harper D R and Dale J J (1985) Chronic ulceration of the leg: extent of the problem and provision of care. *British Medical Journal*, **290**: 1855–1856.

Coleridge-Smith P D, Thomas P, Scurr J H and Dormandy J A (1988) Causes of venous ulceration: a new hypothesis. *British Medical Journal*, **296**: 1726–1727.

Dale J J, Callam M J, Ruckley C V, Harper D R and Berrey P N (1983) Chronic ulcers of the leg: a study of prevalence in a Scottish community. *Health Bulletin*, **41**: 310–314.

3

The Epidemiology of Leg Ulcers

INTRODUCTION

The epidemiology of venous ulcers addresses a variety of questions. We need to know the size of the problem in the population and whether this is changing, for the planning of health care resources. The identification of risk factors is clearly important, primarily to suggest the scope for preventative measures. Risk factors may be suggested by international and temporal comparisons of descriptive data, but one needs to be careful of spurious associations that arise from comparisons in heterogeneous populations. Risk factors are best assessed using case control studies.

PREVALENCE AND INCIDENCE

The description of the level of disease in the population is commonly expressed by two measures. Prevalence, the proportion of the population with the disease at a particular point in time, is determined by cross-sectional surveys of the population. Incidence, the rate of occurrence of new cases of a disease, is obtained from longitudinal population studies. In a condition such as venous ulcers, recurrent cases may be misclassified as incident cases. The most useful measure of temporal change is a change in incidence, since this implies changes in risk factors. Changes in prevalence are much more difficult to interpret, since they include components of both incidence, recurrence and resolution or cure. Also, to be confident of real changes in prevalence, the cross-sectional surveys must be truly representative and the survey methods of ascertainment unchanged. This caution also applies to the comparison of regional or international differences in prevalence, e.g. differences in venous ulcer prevalence between Switzerland and England, based on data obtained from a study of chemical workers in Basel (Widmer, 1978) and a population survey in Scotland (Callam et al, 1985). Real differences in prevalence between these two countries could not be inferred, since a working population is not representative of the general population for many factors, including age, gender and health.

To estimate prevalence and incidence, cases and populations must be defined.

The definition of a venous ulcer should exclude foot ulcers, which are primarily associated with diabetes, and methods of assessment should identify the small proportion of leg ulcers which are arterial. Cases are usually defined as current or active; however restricting the interest only to current cases may underestimate the overall burden to the health services, due to the recurrence rate of healed ulcers, and the definition could include any recent ulcers. Prevalence of a *history* of ulceration is rather imprecise, and may inflate the older, age-specific prevalence rates, since prevalence rates of a history will cumulate with age. The population sampled should be representative of the population being described.

A variety of methods have been used to estimate venous ulcer prevalence.

1. The optimum method is to estimate prevalence from a random or total sample of the 'at risk' population, using a standardized clinical examination. The disadvantages of this approach are that very large surveys are needed for conditions with a relatively low prevalence. One study focused on a 1 in 20 random sample of the population aged over 25 years, in Skaraborg, Sweden, and had a 70 per cent response rate to an invitation to attend for a health check (Hallbook, 1988). Sixty two ulcers were found in the sample of 5631 subjects, giving an overall prevalence of 11/1000, rising to 20/1000 in subjects aged over 60. At younger ages (below 40), ulcers were unusual, with a sharp rise in prevalence in both men and women after this age, and thereafter becoming more common in women than men.

The Tecumseh population study of 4467 subjects aged over 20, in which examination of the legs was a part of a health survey for many conditions, yielded only 13 venous ulcers (11 healed and only two active), three in men and 10 in women (Coon et al, 1973). The prevalence rates in the over 60s was 9.8 per 1000. Including the population data from younger subjects in the sample (who had no cases) gave an overall prevalence rate of 2.9 per 1000 (95 per cent confidence limits from 1.6 to 4.9 per 1000).

A large screening study in Western Australia found 259 chronic leg ulcers in a population of 238 000, giving an overall prevalence of 1.1/1000 (Baker et al, 1992).

2. An alternative method of estimating prevalence in the community is the use of questionnaires to survey the population. This is cheaper than using clinical examination, but the results are dependent on the response rates to the questionnaire and the validity of the questionnaire. Some numerical estimates of how good the questionnaire is can be obtained by calculating the **sensitivity** (the proportion of true cases that are questionnaire positive) and **specificity** (the proportion of true negatives that are questionnaire negative).

Three recent studies have used this method (Dale et al, 1983; Henry, 1986; Wright et al, 1992). The Lothian and Forth Valley study was a pilot study of 800 subjects aged 65–80, on the list of one general practitioner (Dale et al, 1983); the study in Ireland appended the questionnaire to a regular EEC consumer study based on a national random sample of households (ages above 25) (Henry, 1986); and the Riverside study (Wright et al, 1992) used a random sample of approximately 2000 subjects aged 35–70 years on the list of three general practitioners in the Riverside district of West London. The response rates were moderately respectable; 64 per cent in the Riverside study, 72 per cent in the Lothian and

Forth Valley study and were not given for the Irish study. The questionnaires all provided a definition of leg or foot ulcer, with two studies asking for a history (Dale et al, 1983; Wright et al, 1992) and the Irish survey for current ulcers (Henry, 1986). The proportion of questionnaire positives varied from 1.5 per cent in Ireland (ages above 25) and 4.7 per cent (ages above 65), to 4 per cent in Riverside (ages 35–70) and 6 per cent in Lothian and Forth Valley (65–80).

The Lothian and Forth Valley study used two methods to estimate the false positive and false negative rates. False positives were ascertained either by a clinical examination of the patient or, as only 40 per cent responded to the invitation for examination, from the medical records. There was no confirmation in 13 out of 33 who said they had ulcers on the questionnaire, giving a false positive rate of 39 per cent (table 3.1). Most of the patients giving false positive responses had misunderstood 'leg ulcers' for any ulcers or any skin condition of the leg. False negatives were ascertained by sending the questionnaire to 100 subjects known to have clinically confirmed ulcers. Using the data from this survey, the false negative rate may be estimated (shown in parentheses). The false negative rate was 5 per cent, giving a high specificity of 98 per cent. Sensitivity was low at 34 per cent. The overall predictive value of the questionnaire to ascertain cases was 61 per cent. Adjusting for the false positive rate reduced the estimates of prevalence of a history of venous ulcers in the age group 65–80 to 36/1000. The data from Ireland suggests much higher prevalence of current cases (47/1000), but may be biased both by the response rate and the false positive rate.

Table 3.1 Questionnaire survey on venous ulcers

Questionnaire	Medical records		Total
	+	−	
+	20	13	33
−	38	659	697
Total	58	672	730

Sensitivity = 34%; specificity = 98%; predictive value = 61%; false positive = 39%; false negative = 5%.

3. Another method of estimating the prevalence of ulcers has been to use opportunistic surveys of subjects. Prevalence rates derived from these studies are often unreliable as indicators of the community prevalence since the patients are unrepresentative of the background population.

Thus the prevalence of a current or past venous ulcer in 1755 adult patients (75 per cent women) attending a health centre in Brazil was 36/1000 overall; in the age group 60–69, 30/1000 in men and 100/1000 in women, and with rates as high as 160/1000 in the over 70s (Maffeii et al, 1986). These very high estimates are only partly accounted for by the case definition, which included a history of ulceration.

Conversely, the study on venous disorders by the Basel group, undertaken in 4529 workers in the local chemical factories, may have underestimated the prevalence, since few elderly were included (Widmer, 1978). Moreover, the population studied was predominantly male (83 per cent) and older women (at the highest risk) represented only 1 per cent of the sample. The definition of an ulcer in this study included those active or healed. There were few cases before the age of 45, with rates rising from 7/1000 in men and 4/1000 in women aged 45–54; the corresponding figures for men and women respectively for other ages were 14/1000 and 35/1000 for those aged 55–64; and 29/1000 and 48/1000 for those aged over 65.

4. A method of obtaining a good yield of cases without the resources entailed in a huge survey is to ascertain all cases receiving treatment in a defined area with a known population structure. This restricts the definition of prevalence to current cases and relies heavily on complete ascertainment of cases. Errors in the estimate of numbers of cases can occur: by missing cases, for example, some patients may be treated at a specialist centre outside the region or may not be known to health personnel; alternatively extra cases from outside the population at risk may be included. Errors in the population denominator are most likely to occur in the elderly, who since the census date may have died or moved to residential homes or to live with their families outside the catchment area and therefore artificially appear in the denominator but not in the numerator. Another problem relates to the extrapolation of estimates, however precise, since the region surveyed may differ in some risk factor and have higher or lower rates than the national. Clearly this is not an issue in planning resources for that particular region.

Nonetheless, the relative strengths of this method are shown by two studies in the UK: the Lothian and Forth Valley study in Scotland (Callam et al, 1985), and the Northwick Park study in North West London (Cornwall et al, 1986). A total of 1477 cases were ascertained in Lothian and Forth Valley, in a population of approximately 1 million, during the period 1981–1982, and 357 cases in Northwick Park, in a population of 198 000, also surveyed in 1981–1982. The estimates are remarkably consistent in these two studies. The overall prevalence in the adult population of current ulcers was 1.5 per 1000 in Lothian and Forth Valley, and 1.8 per 1000 in Northwick Park. The prevalence in the younger age groups was very low (less than 1/1000 under the age of 50); the data are shown only for men and women over this age (see table 3.2). In both studies, prevalence continued to rise with age, even in the elderly, with estimates of as many as 20 per 1000 in women over the age of 80 with venous ulcers.

Table 3.2 Prevalence of venous ulcers based on case ascertainment by health personnel in two UK studies (rates per 1000)

Study	Age group				
Lothian	55–64	65–74	75–84	85+	overall (18+)
men	1.7	3.4	5.1	7.2	1.5
women	3.1	6.3	11.6	18.9	
Northwick Park	51–60	61–70	71–80	80+	overall (18+)
	1	3	7	20	1.8

A Swedish study used a similar method of case ascertainment (Nelzen et al, 1991). A total of 827 active leg ulcer cases were found in a population of 270 800, giving an overall prevalence of 3/1000. In order to verify the reports of ulcers, a sample of 415 patients were invited to a clinical examination. The response rate was 96 per cent. Of those who attended, only four patients did not meet the criteria for an active ulcer. Thus the estimate of prevalence was little changed. The prevalence rate from the Swedish Study was three times higher than that for the two UK studies and caution is needed in interpreting this result. The overall prevalence may conceal substantial differences in the age structure of the populations. Age specific prevalence data from the Swedish study are given in table 3.3. At ages 55–64 and ages 65–74 the rates are similar in the Lothian and Forth Valley and Swedish population. From the age of 75 the rates appear considerably higher in the Swedish population. However, the ages of 166 patients in the Lothian and Forth Valley study were not known and any resultant bias may account for the discrepancy between the two countries in the oldest age group.

Table 3.3 Age specific prevalence of active leg ulcers, Skaraborg County, West Sweden (Nelzen et al, 1991)

Age group	Men (rate per 1000)	Women (rate per 1000)
<25	0.008	0.022
25–34	0.11	0.18
35–44	0.2	0.21
45–54	1.08	0.69
55–64	2.7	3.4
65–74	4.9	8.1
75–84	15.6	23.8
85+	33.3	34.5

The prevalence rates are presented separately for men and women in the Lothian and Forth Valley and Swedish data, and show an excess rate for women compared to men at all ages in the elderly.

Comparing the prevalence rates in the 65–80 year olds of 36/1000 for a history of ulcers (Dale et al, 1983), and the prevalence rates of 7/1000 of current ulcers in the same case ascertainment study, suggests that less than a quarter of ulcers are open at any one time. Incidence data is much more difficult to obtain and requires longitudinal follow-up of a population using the same methods to ascertain cases, and a knowledge of the false negative rate. To date there are no incidence studies published.

BURDEN ON HEALTH SERVICES

The UK studies showed that most ulcers are looked after by the general practitioner: 67 per cent in the Lothian and Forth Valley study (Callam et al, 1985), 78 per cent in the Northwick Park study (Cornwall et al, 1986). The principal carer was the district nurse, even when patients were attending hospital outpatient clinics (30 per cent) in the Lothian and Forth Valley study. In the Northwick Park study, 69 per cent of ulcers were dressed at home, 48 per cent by the district nurse and 21 per cent by a relative or the patient (usually with poor instruction and supervision). Forty seven per cent of patients never took a bath, to avoid wetting the ulcer. The authors also considered that the treatment was inadequate in 68 per cent: 17 per cent wearing no support and 51 per cent a single bandage only. The Irish questionnaire survey found that 60 per cent of patients reporting ulcers were not receiving health care (Henry, 1986). This high figure is probably only in part accounted for by a high false positive rate.

The district nurse-time surveyed in the Lothian and Forth Valley study was considerable: 22 per cent of patients were treated daily, 16 per cent twice a week, 28 per cent three times a week and 26 per cent every week (Dale, 1984; Callam et al, 1987a). Treatment times varied from 15 to 45 minutes and to this should be added the 25 per cent of district nurse time spent in travelling to the patients' homes.

The Lothian and Forth Valley study obtained detailed information on the clinical history of a sample of 600 of the 1477 leg ulcer cases identified in the original study (Callam et al, 1987b). Twenty two per cent of patients maintained their ulcer had started before the age of 40 and 40 per cent before the age of 50. This led to very long duration periods estimated for the chronic disease, with 45 per cent reporting episodes of ulceration for more than 10 years. Half of current ulcers were reported open for more than 9 months, 20 per cent had not healed after 2 years and 8 per cent were still open after 5 years. Many ulcers were recurrent (67 per cent). Similar figures were reported by the Northwick Park study: 50 per cent of ulcers had been present for more than one year.

Moreover, the health care burden is increased by many patients having ulcers on both legs: 38 per cent in the Lothian and Forth Valley study, and 16 per cent in the Northwick Park study.

RISK FACTORS

Demographic

All studies show a consistent effect of age and sex. At younger ages, women appear to have a lower prevalence than men, but the rate rises faster than in men around middle age, leading to an approximately two-fold excess in older women. Although popularly believed to be mainly a disease associated with social classes IV and V, there is little evidence to support this. A sample of 600 of the 1477 leg ulcer cases identified in the Lothian and Forth Valley study were interviewed about their employment; social class was coded using the Registrar General's classification (Callam et al, 1988). Fifty four per cent were retired and 25 per cent were housewives. The distribution of social class in the sample was compared with that in Lothian and Forth Valley, and was found to be similar. However the duration of an ulcer problem appeared class-related, with more patients in social classes I and II reporting ulcer duration of less than 5 years (54 per cent), compared with social class III (46 per cent) and social classes IV and V (30 per cent). The main reservation in accepting the evidence from this study is that the sample of 600 were not randomly selected but were the first 600 to attend for interview. The response rate was not given.

Medical History

Sixty eight per cent of the 600 patients interviewed and examined in the Lothian and Forth Valley study had varicose veins, 21 per cent arterial insufficiency, 17 per cent a history of hypertension, 8.5 per cent rheumatoid disease and 5.5 per cent diabetes (Ruckley et al, 1982). Half of those with arterial insufficiency also had evidence of chronic venous insufficiency (Callam et al, 1987c). Nearly half were obese (15 per cent over ideal weight), and 32 per cent had severe limitation of the ankle joint. Seventeen per cent were chairbound and 2 per cent bedbound.

In the Northwick Park study, 19 per cent had symptoms of intermittent claudication, 32 per cent a history of some form of arthritis and 5 per cent diabetes. Five per cent were completely immobile (Cornwall et al, 1986). A clinical examination on 100 subjects from their sample of 357 was also completed: 43 per cent had superficial vein incompetence, and 38 per cent had popliteal valve incompetence. Thirty one per cent had ischaemia, and this was in conjunction with a venous defect in a large proportion. Seventy per cent of patients with a history of intermittent claudication had ischaemia. The proportion of legs with ischaemia rose with age, from none in patients under 60 years to 50 per cent in patients over 80.

The problem in interpreting these data is the lack of controls. Arthritis, diabetes, hypertension and venous incompetence are common conditions, especially in the elderly. The Tecumseh study reported an overall prevalence of varicose veins in the adult population of 130/1000 in men and 260/1000 in women (Coon et al, 1973). The corresponding figures for the over 60 age groups were 500/1000 and 750/1000. The 60 per cent figures for varicose veins in the Lothian and Forth Valley study are approximately those that might be expected in the background population. Moreover, even if an increase in these conditions was found in the ulcer population, it may be due to the fact that these conditions are also due to an associated risk factor.

Deep Vein Thrombosis (DVT)

DVT has frequently been cited as a predisposing factor to venous insufficiency and ulcers. In the Tecumseh study, the presence of varicose veins, oedema, stasis changes and venous ulcers was assessed in subjects with a history of DVT (Coon et al, 1973). Seventy two per cent had some vein-related condition; primarily varicose veins. Eighteen per cent had stasis changes, but only 3 per cent an active or healed ulcer. Conversely, 30 per cent of the venous ulcer group had a history of DVT. Other studies have reported deep venous insufficiency occurring in up to 50 per cent of patients after DVT and influenced by factors such as increasing age and length of follow-up (Gjores, 1956; Lindhagen et al, 1984). When the 'at risk' leg was considered in patients with a history of DVT, the incidence of venous insufficiency was found to be similar in both legs, suggesting other predisposing factors (Lindhagen et al, 1985). Obstruction of the deep veins was however more common in legs with a history of DVT.

The Tecumseh study gave the prevalence of a history of DVT as 10/1000 in adult men and 40/1000 in adult women, with a two fold increase in prevalence in the over 60's. In men, the incidence rate increased with age, but in women the rate rose rapidly in young women, with high levels maintained into old age. A history suggestive of DVT was reported in 8 per cent of patients with leg ulcers in the Northwick Park study, which is probably higher than expected on the basis of population prevalence.

However, many episodes of DVT may be asymptomatic and consequently not reported by the patient. Recent use of techniques such as fibrinogen scanning and venography suggests that the post-operative incidence of DVT is high with figures of 30 per cent in Europe and 16 per cent in North America of DVT after general surgery (Hirsh et al, 1986).

SUMMARY

This chapter highlights some of the pitfalls in ascertaining the occurrence and risk factors for venous ulceration. There is probably adequate good quality research on the prevalence of venous ulcers in the UK and more attention should be focused on risk factors. Thus a good estimate of the overall prevalence of active venous ulcers in the UK adult population is around 1.5/1000. Prevalence rises with age, and is higher in women than in men such that in the elderly (over 65) the rates are 4/1000 in men and 9/1000 in women. The prevalence of chronic venous ulcers may be three to four times greater. Risk factors for venous insufficiency have attracted a reasonable amount of research interest, with age, female gender and parity identified consistently as risk factors. However, little attention has been paid to the prediction of risk for ulceration in the population with venous disease or in the assessment of the magnitude of the risk factors for venous ulcers in properly controlled studies. The role of DVT needs clarification.

References

Baker S R, Stacey M C, Singh G, Hoskin S E and Thompson P J (1992) Aetiology of chronic leg ulcers. *European Journal of Vascular Surgery*, **6**: 245–251.
Callam M J, Ruckley C V, Harper D R and Dale J J (1985) Chronic ulceration of the leg: extent of the problem and provision of care. *British Medical Journal*, **290**: 1855–1856.
Callam M J, Dale J J, Harper D R and Ruckley C V (1987a) *Lothian & Forth Valley Leg Ulcer Study*. Hawick: Buccleuch Printers.
Callam M J, Harper D R, Dale J J and Ruckley C V (1987b) Chronic ulcer of the leg: clinical history. *British Medical Journal*, **294**: 1389–1391.
Callam M J, Harper D R, Dale J J and Ruckley C V (1987c) Arterial disease in chronic

leg ulceration: an underestimated hazard? Lothian and Forth Valley leg ulcer study. *British Medical Journal*, **294**: 929–931.

Callam M J, Harper D R, Dale J J and Ruckley C V (1988) Chronic leg ulceration: socio-economic aspects. *Scottish Medical Journal*, **33**: 358–360.

Coon W W, Willis P W III and Keller J B (1973) Venous thromboembolism and other venous disease in the Tecumseh community health study. *Circulation*, **48**: 839–846.

Cornwall J V, Dore C J and Lewis J D (1986) Leg ulcers: epidemiology and aetiology. *British Journal of Surgery*, **73**: 693–696.

Dale J (1984) Knee deep in leg ulcers. *Journal of District Nursing*, **2**(8): 4–8.

Dale J J, Callam M J, Ruckley C V, Harper D R and Berrey P N (1983) Chronic ulcers of the leg: a study of prevalence in a Scottish community. *Health Bulletin (Edinburgh)*, **41**: 310–314.

Gjores J E (1956) The incidence of venous thrombosis and its sequelae in certain districts of Sweden. *Acta Chirurgica Scandinavica Supplementum (Stockholm)*, **26**, 3–89.

Hallbook T (1988) Leg ulcer epidemiology. *Acta Chirurgica Scandinavica Supplementum (Stockholm)*, **544**: 17–20.

Henry M (1986) Incidence of varicose ulcers in Ireland. *Irish Medical Journal*, **79**(3): 65–67.

Hirsh H, Hull R D and Raskob G E (1986) Epidemiology and pathogenesis of venous thrombosis. *Journal of the American College of Cardiology*, **8**: 104–111.

Lindhagen A, Berqvist D and Hallbook T (1984) Deep venous insufficiency after post-operative thrombosis diagnosed with ^{125}I-fibrinogen uptake test. *British Journal of Surgery*, **71**: 511–515.

Lindhagen A, Berqvist D, Hallbook T and Efsing H O (1985) Venous function five to eight years after clinically suspected deep venous thrombosis. *Acta Medica Scandinavica (Stockholm)*, **217**: 389–395.

Maffeii F H A, Magaldi C, Pinho S Z, Lastoria S, Pinho W, Yoshida W B and Rollo H A (1986) Varicose veins and chronic venous insufficiency in Brazil: prevalence among 1,755 inhabitants of a country town. *International Journal of Epidemiology*, **15**: 210–217.

Nelzen O, Berqvist D, Lindehagen A and Hallbook T (1991) Chronic leg ulcers: an under-estimated problem in primary health care among elderly patients. *Journal of Epidemiology and Community Health*, **45**: 184–187.

Ruckley, C V, Dale J J, Callam M J and Harper D R (1982) Causes of chronic leg ulcer. *Lancet*, **ii**, 615–616.

Widmer L K (1978) *Peripheral Venous Disorders: Prevalence and Sociomedical Importance*. Bern: Hans Huber.

Wright D D I, Franks P J, Monro C, Stirling J, Fletcher A E, Bulpitt C J and McCollum C N (1992) Prevalence of venous disease in West London. *European Journal of Surgery*, **158**: 143–147.

4

The Nursing Assessment of
Patients with Leg Ulcers

INTRODUCTION

Surveys have shown that approximately 85 per cent of leg ulcer patients are treated in the community by district nurses and/or general practitioners (Callam et al, 1985). The general practitioner may write the prescription, but leave the choice and frequency of treatment to his nursing colleagues. It is therefore important that nurses generally, and particularly those working in the community and in nursing homes, are taught to recognise the different types of ulcer.

This chapter will describe those methods of nursing assessment which are essential before any decision regarding management is made. The most successful nurse practitioners should be able to carry out a detailed assessment, and be aware when medical advice should be sought.

Accurate assessment is the key to successful treatment of any patient and patients with leg ulcers are no exception.

In previous chapters we have learned that there are different types of leg ulcers, and it is extremely important that nurses are aware of the cause and underlying pathology before making any decision regarding treatment.

Accurate diagnosis is the key to successful treatment; as whilst purely venous ulcers require compression bandaging to improve venous return, it would be extremely dangerous to apply compression therapy to an ischaemic leg.

THE ASSESSMENT

All findings of the assessment should be recorded (for an example of an assessment form see figure 4.1).

The assessment should begin by concentrating on the patient as a whole. The patient's age, sex and parity are all relevant, as many leg ulcer sufferers are elderly females, some of whom may have developed deep vein thrombosis or varicose veins during pregnancy.

The patient's occupation (or past occupation if retired) may also contribute to the ulcer pathology, especially jobs where standing is prolonged, such as hairdressers and shop assistants. Nurses should also be aware of their patients' living

EXAMPLE ASSESSMENT FORM

PATIENT'S NAME   HOSP NO

ADDRESS

TEL NO   AGE
                      SEX M:F

GP:

DATE ☐☐☐☐☐☐

OCCUPATION: _____

PARITY: (if appropriate) _____

SMOKER: Current ☐

      Former ☐

MOBILITY: Walks freely   ☐

      Walks with aids ☐

Ankle____cms. Gaiter____cms.

Calf____cms.

Height____cms ft.____ins.____

Weight____kgs. st.____lbs.____

Urine: Protein____   Glucose____

Blood____   Other____

Blood Pressure____

Previous Medical History: please tick boxes where appropriate,

M.I. _____	☐	Pulmonary Embolism	☐
C.V.A. _____	☐	Previous D.V.T.	☐
T.I.A. _____	☐	Thrombophlebitis	☐
Claudication _____	☐	Lower Leg Fractures	☐
Previous Arterial Surgery _____	☐	Previous V.V. Surgery	☐
Diabetes _____	☐	Previous Sclerotherapy	☐
Arthritis _____	☐	V.V.'s present	☐
Leg Oedema _____	☐	Lipodermatosclerosis	☐

Record Allergies _____

_____

Record Present Medication _____

Fig 4.1 Assessment form

ULCER HISTORY

		Right Leg	Left Leg
Duration of present ulcer (months)		☐	☐
Onset of first ulcer (years)		☐	☐
Number of episodes		☐	☐
LEVEL:	Calf	☐	☐
	Gaiter	☐	☐
	Foot	☐	☐
ASPECT:	Anterior	☐	☐
	Posterior	☐	☐
	Medial	☐	☐
	Lateral	☐	☐
	Medial and lateral	☐	☐
	Circumferential	☐	☐
Size – in mms		☐	☐
APPEARANCE:	Slough	☐	☐
	Granulating	☐	☐
	Epithelialising	☐	☐
DEPTH:	Superficial	☐	☐
	Deep	☐	☐
SKIN:	Normal	☐	☐
	Dry eczema	☐	☐
	Wet eczema	☐	☐
	Maceration	☐	☐
	Cellulitis	☐	☐
ANKLE MOVEMENT:	Full	☐	☐
	Restricted	☐	☐
	Fixed	☐	☐
PEDAL PULSES PALPABLE:	DPP	☐	☐
	PTP	☐	☐
API (Arm/Ankle Pressure Index if available)		☐	☐

Summary of Causes – please circle

Venous	Arterial	Arthritic	Vasculitic
Diabetic	Obesity	Trauma	Malignancy
		Frailty	Poor
			Mobility

Other...

conditions; cold, damp rooms may encourage elderly patients to sit too close to the fire, causing scorching of the skin or 'Grannie's tartan'. Nights spent sitting upright in a chair, with legs dependent, rather than retiring to a cold bedroom, are a major cause of oedematous legs.

The patient's height and weight should be measured and recorded, as many leg ulcer sufferers are grossly overweight (Callam and Ruckley, 1992), resulting in reduced mobility and inducing strain on the ulcerated limb. The level of mobility should also be assessed. This facilitates the setting of realistic exercise goals and enables any improvement or deterioration in mobility to be detected. The nurse should record whether the patient walks freely or needs to use a walking stick or Zimmer frame.

Poor diet, common in the elderly, can hinder the healing process, whilst smoking is of special significance in patients with ischaemic ulcers, as it exacerbates the arterial constriction.

Ankle joint mobility should be noted, as limitation of ankle movement will lead to poor utilisation of the calf muscle pump and exercise is important to improve venous return. The patient's level of awareness may help or hinder progress; the confused or demented elderly person living alone may require more frequent visits from the nurse, and this should be taken into account when assessing the patient's needs and planning care.

The patient's past medical history will provide many clues as to the underlying cause of the ulcer. A previous history of myocardial infarction, intermittent claudication, strokes or transient ischaemic attacks, diabetes or rheumatoid arthritis are all indicative of arterial disease. A history of arterial surgery (e.g. coronary artery bypass graft) also indicates the presence of arterial disease which may be the cause of ulceration or an important complicating factor. This information may be gleaned from the patient at interview or from the patient's medical notes if these are available.

Urinalysis for glycosuria should be undertaken to eliminate diabetes and the patient's joints examined for any signs of arthritis. Rheumatoid arthritis can be confirmed or eliminated by sending a blood sample to the laboratory for serology. Leg ulcers associated with rheumatoid arthritis are often slow to heal, and prolonged steroid therapy weakens the skin and delays the healing process.

Blood pressure should be recorded routinely as it contributes to the clinical picture. Hypertension is of little significance to the ulcer pathology, but may be another indication of cardiovascular disease and ischaemic ulceration.

The whole leg should be examined carefully. Eczema and staining of the skin around the ulcer are an indication that venous disease is present; induration and ankle flare (distension of the network of small veins on the medial aspect of the foot just below the malleolus) are sure signs of chronic venous insufficiency (see plate 1).

Varicose veins may be present and although brown staining and discolouration of the skin do not occur in association with purely arterial ulcers, all these signs may be present in ulcers of mixed aetiology (see table 4.1).

An ischaemic foot/leg looks white or bluish and feels cold to the touch. Shiny, hairless skin, poor capillary filling and night pain (relieved by hanging the leg over

Table 4.1   Factors associated with venous ulcers

Eczema
Staining of the skin around the ulcer
Induration and ankle flare
Varicose veins
Oedema
Previous deep vein thrombosis
History of pulmonary emboli
Previous leg fracture
Palpable foot pulse
History of varicose vein surgery or sclerotherapy

the edge of the bed) are all indicative of ischaemic disease (plate 2). Capillary filling can be assessed by pressing gently on the patient's great toe nail and causing the nailbed to blanche. When the pressure is removed, the colour should return instantly; however, if the leg is ischaemic the colour of the nailbed will take much longer to return to normal. However, it should be noted that both skin colour and capillary filling will be affected by cold, and examination of the legs should be undertaken in a warm room. The factors associated with arterial or mixed aetiology ulcers are summarized in table 4.2.

Table 4.2   Factors associated with arterial/mixed ulcers

History of heart disease
History of stroke
Intermittent claudication
Transient ischaemic attacks
Diabetes
Rheumatoid arthritis
Previous arterial surgery
Foot pulses not palpable
Shiny, hairless skin
Poor capillary filling
White, colourless leg
Cold, bluish foot

Checking the foot pulses is the most important simple test for detecting arterial disease. The dorsalis pedis pulse (DP) is palpable in the midline of the foot, in front of the ankle joint, and the posterior tibial pulse (PTP) behind the medial malleolus (plates 3 and 4). Absent or very weak pulses indicate poor peripheral blood supply and further testing with a Doppler ultrasound flow detector is recommended. Local areas of capillary infarction can cause loss of pigment in the skin, with small pale areas known as 'atrophie blanche' (Shornick et al, 1983).

Some patients have ulcers of mixed aetiology, where venous and arterial disease may be present at the same time. The contributory factors listed in tables 4.1 and 4.2 will help to confirm the diagnosis, but it is very important to ascertain the severity of the ischaemia. Doppler ultrasound may be used to measure the **ankle: brachial pressure index (ABPI)**. This is essential before any decision regarding the management of ulcers with an arterial component can be made (Cameron, 1991). It is important, however, that a diagnosis is not made solely on the result of the Doppler ultrasound examination, which only aids diagnosis. When any uncertainty exists about the diagnosis (e.g. due to difficulty feeling foot pulses or poor capillary filling), Doppler ultrasound will confirm the degree of ischaemia present.

To record the ABPI, the patient should lie flat on a couch and be as relaxed as possible. The sphygmomanometer cuff is secured around the arm, ultrasound gel applied over the brachial pulse and the Doppler probe is held over the pulse. The cuff is inflated until the pulse signal disappears, then the cuff is deflated until the pulse signal returns. The pressure at which the signal returns is the **brachial systolic pressure**.

The **ankle systolic pressure** is obtained by applying the sphygmomanometer cuff just above the ankle (if the ulcer is situated in the gaiter area it should be covered with a non-adherent dressing). The dorsalis pedis or posterior tibial pulse should be found by palpation and whichever gives the best signal used for the measurement. Ultrasound gel should be applied over the site of the pulse and the above procedure repeated to obtain the ankle systolic pressure. If the pulses are not palpable, ultrasound gel should be applied to one of the pulse sites, the probe held over the area and, as the signal is directional, the angle of the head of the probe should be changed until the signal is clearly heard (plate 5). The ankle pressure is divided by the brachial pressure to calculate the ABPI, also called the **resting pressure index (RPI)**.

In normal subjects, the arterial pressure in the leg is the same as or higher than that in the arm, so the ratio of the pressure in the leg to that in the arm is at least 1. If the leg is ischaemic, the systolic pressure at the ankle will be lower than that in the arm and the ratio will be 0.9 or less. An ABPI of less than 0.8 indicates the presence of significant arterial disease. Nurses should be aware, however, that in the presence of severe atherosclerosis it may be difficult to occlude the arteries with a sphygmomanometer cuff due to calcification of the arteries. In these circumstances, very high pressures, suggesting adequate perfusion, may be measured. This could be very misleading. It should also be noted that patients with diabetes may have a normal ABPI; however, high levels of compression are still a risk because of the likelihood of small vessel disease.

The site of the ulcer may be an important indicator of the underlying pathology, and should be recorded. Most venous ulcers occur in the gaiter area (figure 4.2), i.e. the lower third of the leg; the most common site being the medial malleolar area. Ulcers outwith the gaiter area should be treated with caution; ulcers on the foot are usually due to ischaemia or diabetes, whilst ulcers in the calf are usually not due to venous disease either but may be due to vasculitis, especially if the ulcers are small and scattered.

Oedema is a common problem, especially in venous disease, and should be reduced by leg elevation before the application of compression bandaging. However, oedema may also be present in arterial disease and where ulcers are of mixed aetiology, and the cause of oedema must be evaluated for each patient. Oedema may be due to immobility, limb dependence or a fixed ankle joint, but a history of heart or kidney failure must be borne in mind when deciding how to reduce oedema. Gross lymphoedema resulting from obstructed lymph vessels is a rare cause of ulceration. Oedema associated with arterial or diabetic ulcers tends to be more localised.

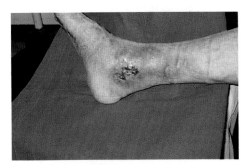

Plate 1   Venous staining, varicose veins and ankle flare

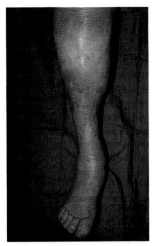

Plate 2   Ischaemic leg with shiny, hairless skin

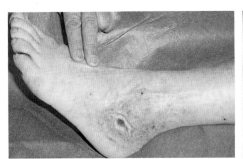

Plate 3   Dorsalis pedis pulse

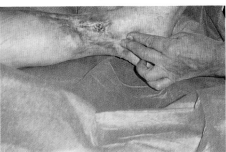

Plate 4   Posterior tibial pulse

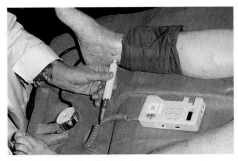

Plate 5   Doppler ultrasound

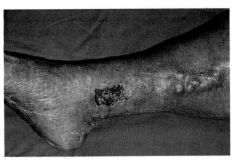

Plate 6   Venous ulcer

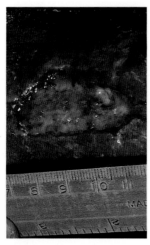

Plate 7 Arterial ulcer

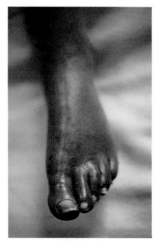

Plate 8 Diabetic foot with ulcerated toe

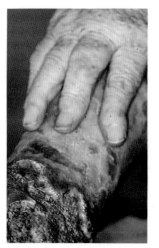

Plate 9 Rheumatoid ulcer

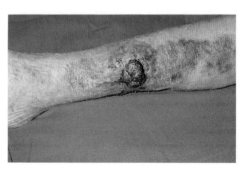

Plate 10 Malignant ulcer

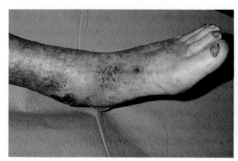

Plate 11 Skin damage on the foot due to pressure

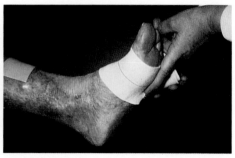

Plate 12 Bandaging the foot

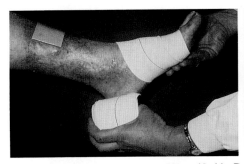
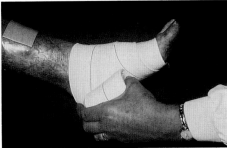

Plates 13, 14 Bandaging the foot

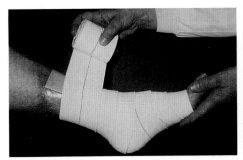
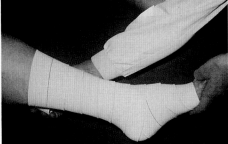

Plates 15, 16 Spiral bandaging of the leg

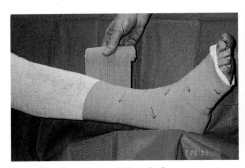
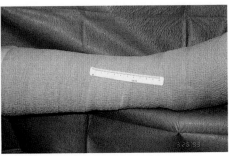

Plate 17 Figure of eight bandaging

Plate 18 Measuring bandage overlap

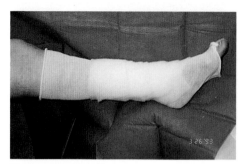

Plate 19 Padding the gaiter

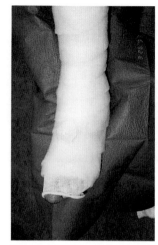

Plate 20 Foam protecting the foot

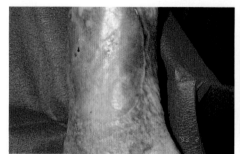

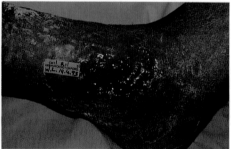

Plate 21 Skin damage at the edge of a dressing   **Plate 22** A leg ulcer surrounded by stasis eczema

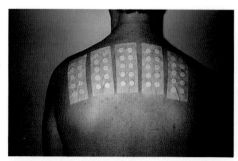

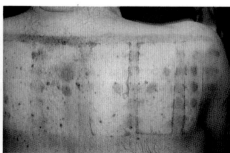

Plate 23 Test strips applied to a patient's back   **Plate 24** A positive patch test

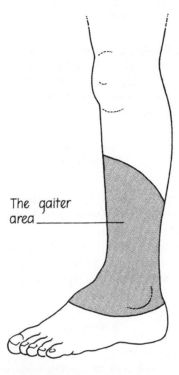

Fig 4.2 Position of gaiter area

The pain associated with leg ulcers can be very severe and is generally less of a problem with venous than arterial ulcers; however, pain in itself is not a diagnostic feature. Arterial ulcers are often painful at night when the legs are elevated, so patients who prefer to sleep in a chair or with their legs dangling out of bed almost certainly have an arterial component to their ulcer. Diabetic ulcers can also be very painful, but neuropathy may reduce the pain sensation in some patients.

Finally the appearance of the ulcer itself may be a guide to diagnosis if used in conjunction with the knowledge already gleaned from the general assessment, but the appearance alone should not dictate the diagnosis (see chapter 2—The aetiology of leg ulceration). Venous ulcers tend to be shallow, well vascularized and situated in the gaiter area with associated signs of venous disease such as ankle flare and varicose veins (see plate 6).

Arterial ulcers are usually paler in appearance, often sloughy and necrotic and may be situated in any part of the lower leg or foot. They may have a punched out look and more depth than venous ulcers. Arterial ulcers are usually very slow to heal (plate 7).

Diabetic ulcers are usually found on the foot, often over bony prominences, e.g. the bunion area of the foot or under the metatarsal heads. Like arterial ulcers they usually have a sloughy or necrotic appearance and are often caused by pressure from footwear, particularly where peripheral neuropathy has anaesthetized the foot (plate 8).

Rheumatoid ulcers may be identified by the presence of arthritic joints. The ulcer often has a shelf-like appearance at the edge, and is usually slow to heal (plate 9). However, it should also be noted that patients with rheumatoid arthritis may also develop ulcers associated with venous disease.

Malignant ulcers often have a rolled edge and an extreme amount of granulation tissue, which will increase rather than reduce in size in spite of diligent care. This type of ulcer is very rare (plate 10).

SUMMARY

- Accurate assessment of the patient with leg ulceration is vital.
- Patients with significant arterial disease must be identified.
- Checking for foot pulses is essential.
- Doppler ultrasound will confirm or exclude the presence of arterial disease.
- The nurse should be aware of the more rare causes of leg ulceration.
- Where there is any doubt, medical advice should be sought.

References

Callam M J, Ruckley C V, Harper D R and Dale J J (1985) Chronic ulceration of the leg: extent of the problem and provision of care. *British Medical Journal*, **240**: 1855–1856.

Callam M J and Ruckley C V (1992) Chronic venous insufficiency and leg ulcers. In: *Surgical Management of Vascular Disease*, eds Ruckley C V, Bell P R F and Jamieson C W, p. 1281. Philadelphia: W B Saunders.

Cameron J (1991) Using Doppler to diagnose leg ulcers. *Nursing Standard*, 5(40): 25–27.

Shornick J K, Nicholes B K, Bergstresser P R and Gilliam J N (1983) Idiopathic atrophie blanche. *Journal of the American Academy of Surgery*, **8**: 792.

5

Topical Applications in Leg
Ulcer Management

INTRODUCTION

The Department of Health Strategy for Nursing (1989) proposed that:

"All clinical practice should be founded on up-to-date information and research findings; practitioners should be encouraged to identify the needs and opportunities for research presented by their work."

The responsibility of individual nurses to be aware of research findings is never so important as in the field of wound care, and leg ulcer management specifically, where nurses are responsible for making most of the treatment decisions (McIntosh, 1979).

This chapter will explore the use of topical applications such as lotions and dressings in leg ulcer management. Decision-making, and particularly product choice in wound care should be guided by research findings; however, it is important that research findings are interpreted in the light of the rigour with which the original research was conducted. For a more comprehensive discussion of how to review research relating to the evidence of effectiveness of therapies, the reader is referred to the excellent chapter 'Deciding on the best therapy' in the book *Clinical Epidemiology: A Basic Science for Clinical Medicine* (Sackett et al, 1991).

Each piece of research included in this chapter has been critically evaluated. It is also important, when reviewing the research evidence relating to the effectiveness of therapeutic interventions, to include as great a proportion as possible of **all** the relevant studies which have been done. To facilitate achievement of this objective, *MEDLINE* has been searched from the year of its inception (1966) to March 1993, by 'exploding' the Medical Subject Heading (MeSH) **LEG ULCER** for all its subheadings, and by searching with the text terms **leg ulcer** and **varicose ulcer**. Citations were also cross-referenced and papers from conference proceedings included.

WOUND CARE RESEARCH

There are a number of indicators which we look for when we are faced with the decision of choosing one dressing or lotion above another. The first one is likely to be, 'Does the product speed up wound healing?'. However this is not the only criterion. Other questions such as 'How often does the product need to be used/changed?', 'Does it have any side effects and if so are they common?', 'Is it comfortable for the patient?', 'Is it easy to use?' are equally important. Although all except the first question can be answered in a study which just examines the product of interest in a group of patients, without a comparison or 'control' product, it is far more meaningful if any new product is compared to another currently commonly used for the same purpose and this is the only type of clinical research which will be included in this review.

Secondly, within any trial of a product, the play of chance should decide which patients receive the test product and which the control. This avoids bias and is achieved by randomly allocating patients to each group, e.g. by the use of random number tables.

Successful randomization should mean that the patients in each experimental group are similar in relation to those factors such as age, duration and size of ulcers that are likely to affect healing rate. Attempting to match or pair patients between groups for such factors as these is one strategy, but it would only be possible to match patients for those factors *known* to be important. Thus the strongest type of evidence for the effectiveness of any wound care product is that derived from the **randomised controlled trial**. A relatively small number of studies in wound care have adopted this, the best technique for evaluating effectiveness. Indeed, as Fletcher (1992) pronounced at the 1st European Conference on Advances in Wound Management,

"Of even greater concern is the paucity of randomised controlled trials to establish therapeutic efficacy *per se* let alone advantages of competing products."

There are a number of ways in which wound care products, or their components may be evaluated. Studies may be carried out *in vitro* on cell cultures, for example, or wound dressings themselves may be subjected to the laboratory testing of performance. Products may be evaluated on wounds artificially produced in animals or healthy volunteers or on real patients with real wounds.

Laboratory-based studies may examine the effect of a product on cells such as fibroblasts, in cell culture. This so-called *in vitro* research is useful in that it allows the researcher to focus on particular cells and their behaviour in a way which is difficult or impossible in the complete wound module. The *in vitro* method is often the method of choice for very preliminary work and may give us an insight into what **may** happen in the wound in a patient; however, it is important to remember when interpreting such work that the findings of such studies can never be assumed to represent what happens *in vivo*, i.e. in the wound of a patient. Nevertheless, such research is very informative and has contributed greatly to our understanding of what happens when cells of the wound module are exposed to antiseptics, for example (e.g. Lineaweaver et al, 1985).

Another widely-used method for the evaluation of wound care products is the animal model. The pig has been particularly well-studied, as its skin is said to closely resemble that of humans. Animal work allows large numbers of very similar wounds to be studied in closely controlled conditions; indeed it was Winter's early work on pigs which revealed the advantages of moist wound healing (Winter, 1962); however, we can never assume that what happens in a pig wound will happen in a patient, who may be debilitated. Clean, surgically-produced wounds rarely resemble the chronic, unhealing wound. It is also worth noting that no good animal model of the chronic venous ulcer exists.

The most meaningful and unfortunately the most difficult wound healing research to undertake is that involving human subjects. This type of study may involve the use of surgically-produced wounds in human volunteers, e.g. Hinman and Maibach's (1963) study of moist versus dry wound healing in human 'volunteers' in San Quentin prison, or may study clinical wounds, such as in patients with venous leg ulcers. Studies in volunteers are useful for preliminary work, as wounds can be produced which are very similar, and the good health of the volunteers means that disease processes will not interfere with healing and confuse the interpretation of the results. However, the best test of whether a particular dressing is useful in patients with burns or patients with leg ulcers is to look at how it performs in patients with these problems.

REVIEW OF THE WOUND HEALING PROCESS

Chronic open wounds such as leg ulcers and pressure sores heal by secondary intention or 'granulation', rather than primary intention (the means by which a surgical incision heals). Careful studies of the cellular components of wound healing have demonstrated that healing begins with an inflammatory phase, characterised by vasodilatation, increased capillary permeability, complement activation, and polymorphonucleocyte (PMN) and macrophage migration into the wound. PMNs predominate during the first few days of injury; however, they are overshadowed by macrophages by around the fifth day. Macrophages are large, mobile and actively phagocytic; engulfing bacteria and devitalised tissue, and so constituting the body's own system for wound debridement. Importantly, macrophages release chemotactic substances which attract more macrophages and that also result, within days, in the emergence of fibroblasts and endothelial cells. Platelets release platelet-derived growth factor, which is also a potent chemoattractant for fibroblasts and smooth muscle cells. The appearance of fibroblasts and endothelial cells around the fifth day post-injury heralds the 'proliferative phase' (Dyson et al, 1988).

Firboblasts are the 'factory cells' of the wound healing module. They are rich in mitochondria, endoplasmic reticulum and Golgi apparatus essential for protein synthesis. Fibroblasts synthesise collagen and ground substance (proteoglycans and fibronectin) which supports new cells and the fragile capillary buds which appear around this time in the process known as angiogenesis. The endothelial buds become patent and increase the blood supply and hence the oxygen tension of the new tissue. These fragile capillary buds, supported in the collagen matrix, are known as 'granulation tissue'. This granulation tissue is then covered by epithelial cells which migrate across its surface and close the epidermal defect.

Collagen synthesis continues for many months after epithelialisation; however, collagen is also undergoing continual lysis during this time and a delicate balance exists between the two processes. This final phase is known as 'remodelling' or 'maturation', and is associated with an increasing tensile strength of the wound and a decreasing cellularity, and may continue for up to a year.

Very little research has been carried out to investigate the differences between acute and chronic wounds. All studies of the wound healing process have been undertaken on acute wounds, usually in experimental animals; unfortunately there is no good animal model of a venous ulcer. How closely the healing of a chronic wound follows the healing pattern of an acute wound is not clear. The question of what makes a chronic wound 'chronic' is yet to be answered. Nursing notes frequently record comments such as 'healing well' repeatedly for months or years! Detailed biochemical and cellular analysis of the chronic wound module is urgently needed.

MOISTURE AND WOUND HEALING

In 1962, George Winter published his seminal text on the effect of occlusion on wound healing. Winter made experimental wounds in Large-White pigs and covered half with occlusive film whilst half were left exposed to the air. The occluded and hence moist wounds epithelialised twice as fast as those left to form a scab.

The Winter study was subsequently followed up by Hinman and Maibach in 1963 who made experimental wounds in healthy adult male volunteers. Punch biopsies of occluded and exposed wounds made at various time intervals demonstrated more epithelialisation in the occluded wounds. It was also noted that epithelial cells in the exposed wounds grew at right angles to the surface of the wound to find a plane of cleavage (or path of least resistance) under the eschar. Occlusion prevented eschar formation, enabling the epithelium to extend directly across the wound surface.

More recently, Alvarez et al (1983) compared the healing of pig wounds covered with semi-permeable film (Opsite™, Smith & Nephew), occlusive hydrocolloid (Granuflex™, Convatec) and saline soaks, with wounds left exposed. Wounds covered with Opsite and Granuflex™ produced significantly more collagen than air-exposed wounds (although the clinical significance of this increase in collagen is not clear). The wounds covered with Granuflex epithelialised more rapidly than those covered by Opsite or saline-soaks. Granuflex is distinct from the film dressing and saline-soaks in that it does not allow gaseous exchange (although the gaseous permeability of the wet or soiled Granuflex was not measured in this study). Dyson et al (1988) examined what happens at a cellular level during healing in moist and dry conditions. They found more inflammatory cells in the dry wounds at 5 days and a more rapid progression from the inflammatory phase to the proliferative phase of healing in the moist wounds.

THE ROLE OF OXYGEN IN WOUND HEALING

Oxygen is essential for cell metabolism and demand for oxygen is increased by synthetic processes such as those occurring during wound healing. Shortly after injury, the oxygen tension in a wound falls, so that by day 3, the oxygen tension in the dead space of a wound is below 10 mmHg (Hunt et al, 1969). This fall in oxygen tension is accompanied by an increase in the concentration of carbon dioxide and a fall in pH. A low oxygen tension is thought to stimulate fibroblast replication and angiogenesis, and hence the production of granulation tissue (Hunt et al, 1969; Knighton et al, 1981).

Oxygen concentrations have been measured under oxygen-permeable (Opsite) and oxygen-impermeable dressings (Granuflex) in patients with chronic leg ulcers (Varghese et al, 1986). The oxygen tension was very low under the film dressing and zero under Granuflex and it was concluded that both dressings, irrespective of oxygen permeability, create the hypoxic conditions which favour wound healing, although the study did not compare the effects of these dressings on wound healing rates.

In summary, a gradient of oxygen tension from a region of high concentration at the level of the capillary, to low concentrations at the margins of granulation under an occlusive dressing, is thought to stimulate angiogenesis (or granulation) and hence healing.

MICROORGANISMS AND WOUND HEALING

The effect of microorganisms on ulcer healing remains an area of debate. That leg ulcers are usually colonized by bacteria is accepted, and an important distinction should be made between 'colonization' and 'infection'. Skin wounds are almost never sterile due to rapid colonization with skin commensal organisms. Infection is characterized by pain, inflammation, purulent exudate and heat, and the more objective measures of a PMN response and tissue concentrations of organisms in excess of 10^5/g (Hutchinson, 1990).

The influence of bacteria on ulcer healing has been examined in a small number of studies. Eriksson (1985a) and Eriksson et al (1984) found that ulcer healing was not influenced by the presence of bacteria. Gilchrist and Reed (1989) monitored the bacterial flora under Granuflex in 20 venous ulcers and found it to be stable over a 12 week treatment period, with the exception of *Pseudomonas* sp. which were inhibited by the dressing. Unfortunately the study was too small and short-lived to relate colonization, or infection to healing outcome, but 55 per cent of ulcers had healed by 12 weeks. No comparison was made with an oxygen-permeable dressing.

The effect of occlusive dressings on infection rates is controversial. Hinman and Maibach (1963) believed that although a moist environment facilitated wound healing, it may also facilitate the growth of bacteria and hence ultimately mitigate against wound healing. This dialogue was reopened in the 1980s with the advent of occlusive hydrocolloid dressings which are impermeable to oxygen. Fears that the moist and hypoxic environment under a hydrocolloid may encourage bacterial growth, and particularly that of anaerobes, appear to be unfounded. Varghese et al (1986) reported that the wound fluid under the occlusive Granuflex was more acidic than that under an oxygen permeable film and *in vitro* studies showed that this pH retarded bacterial growth. In his review of the microbiology of wound healing, Hutchinson (1990) indicates that infection rates under hydrocolloid dressings are generally reported as lower than those under conventional dressings (2 versus 5 per cent, respectively). He proposes that this decreased wound infection rate is due to a combination of more efficient PMN infiltration under occlusion, coupled with the effective barrier to external bacterial invasion which a hydrocolloid provides. The conclusions of this review appear to have been borne out by publication of preliminary data of a prospective multicentre trial comparing Granuflex alone and with Flamazine™ (Smith & Nephew), and tulle gras in venous ulcers, burns and donor sites. Clinical infection rates were generally low; 5.7 per cent in the group receiving tulle gras dressings, 2.1 per cent in the group receiving Granuflex alone and a zero rate of infection in the group receiving Granuflex plus Flamazine (Hutchinson, 1992).

In conclusion, there is little to recommend the routine swabbing of leg ulcers in the absence of clinical infection, as almost all are colonised. Studies conducted to date have been too small and of too short duration to determine the effect of bacteria on healing rates. It is clear that ulcer healing does occur in the presence of both aerobes and anaerobes. Hydrocolloids do not appear to increase infection rates, but do provide effective barriers to cross-infection.

THE PRESENCE OF DEVITALISED TISSUE

Our knowledge of the physiology of wound healing tells us that the presence of an excess of bacteria and devitalised tissue may prolong the inflammatory phase of wound healing. This hypothesis has never been tested in the clinical situation. Haury et al (1980) inoculated experimental wounds in guinea pigs with soft tissue from other guinea pigs. Contralateral wounds were left uninoculated as controls. The introduction of devitalised soft tissue damaged the host's resistance to infection, whether the introduced tissue was muscle, fat or skin. The authors suggest that leucocytes engaged in eliminating large amounts of devitalised tissue lose the ability to ingest bacteria, a proposal further substantiated by Hohn et al (1977).

Devitalised tissue may be removed surgically/mechanically or by the use of appropriate topical applications including dressings (see below).

BARRIERS TO SUCCESSFUL WOUND HEALING

From our discussion of what is known of the physiology and pathophysiology of wound healing, we can now arrive at a list of barriers to successful ulcer healing (table 5.1).

Table 5.1   Barriers to successful ulcer healing

A dry wound bed
Presence of devitalised tissue/slough
Presence of clinical infection
Poor blood supply/anaemia
Poor nutrition
Venous hypertension

OBJECTIVES OF WOUND MANAGEMENT

The long-term objective of leg ulcer management must be to heal the ulcer, as it has been repeatedly shown that this is possible in the majority of cases. However, our list of barriers to healing helps us to develop short-term objectives for every particular wound and these short-term objectives will greatly assist practitioners to pick suitable dressings from the huge range available (table 5.2). It has been argued that the choice of which dressing to apply to a leg ulcer is largely irrelevant, since when patients with venous ulcers were randomized to receive either Granuflex or NA dressings (Backhouse et al, 1987), or Granuflex, NA or Flamazine cream (Blair et al, 1988a, b) under a standardized four-layer compression bandage system, there was no difference in healing rates. However only small ulcers were eligible for inclusion in these studies (mean ulcer area 3 cm² in the Backhouse study) and it could be argued that the research focused on unproblematic ulcers at such a late stage of healing that there was little likelihood of demonstrating the benefit of one dressing against another.

The achievement of wound care objectives is facilitated by the wide range of preparations available for use; these range from protease enzymes used to debride

Table 5.2   Objectives of wound care

Maintain a moist wound environment without causing maceration
Remove excess wound exudate without drying the wound bed
Remove necrotic tissue and slough
Protect the wound from mechanical damage
Maintain the wound temperature
Protect the wound from the introduction of pathogenic organisms
Control odour
Disturb the wound as little as possible

sloughy wounds, to seaweed-derived alginate dressings capable of absorbing large volumes of exudate. Those lotions and dressings commonly used in leg ulcer management will be discussed in the light of their recommended use and the research evidence for their effectiveness. A summary of the randomized controlled trials of dressings which have been undertaken on patients with leg ulcers appears in table 5.3.

CHEMICAL CLEANSERS, DEBRIDERS AND ANTISEPTICS

INDICATIONS: sloughy, dirty and/or necrotic ulcers.

The Evidence

The widespread use of antiseptics for wound cleansing has greatly diminished over recent years (Dale, 1986). Antiseptics such as the hypochlorites (Eusol, Dakin's, Milton's, Chloramine T, sodium hypochlorite) are not only toxic to bacteria, but also to cells of the healing wound. Kozol et al (1988) showed that Dakin's solution (at concentrations as low as 0.000025 per cent) inhibited leucocyte chemotaxis, and injured endothelial cells and fibroblasts. Lineaweaver et al (1985) demonstrated the toxicity of 1 per cent povidone iodine, 0.25 per cent acetic acid, 0.5 per cent sodium hypochlorite and 3 per cent hydrogen peroxide to cultured human fibroblasts, and all except hydrogen peroxide were also shown to be detrimental to wound healing in a rat model. Brennan and Leaper (1985) used laser doppler flowmetry to demonstrate that Eusol, Chloramine T and 5 per cent povidone iodine stopped blood flow in the new capillaries of the rabbit ear chamber (an established granulating wound model). Vessels shut down by the application of these materials had not reopened even after five days. Saline and 1 per cent povidone iodine had no effect, whilst chlorhexidine had a mild effect. Leaper and Brennan (1986) further reported that chlorhexidine, phenol, hexachlorophene, hydrogen peroxide and povidone iodine are toxic to fibroblasts. Tatnall et al (1987) have shown that exposure of keratinocytes in culture to any one of 3 per cent hydrogen peroxide, 1 per cent cetrimide, 0.5 per cent sodium hypochlorite and 4 per cent povidone iodine for 15 minutes resulted in 100 per cent killing of the cells.

These findings have resulted in calls for the 'banning' of the use of Eusol and other hypochlorites. Nurses are fearful of breaching the UKCC Code of Conduct and even litigation if they use such materials at the behest of members of the medical profession, many of whom still advocate the use of hypochlorites in certain situations. These issues have been reviewed by Tingle (1990). The main question is whether the studies discussed above can be extrapolated to the clinical situation. Most of the studies utilised clean, experimentally produced animal wounds or cell cultures. Cunliffe (1990) argues that bacteria themselves are toxic to fibroblasts and keratinocytes, and advocates the use of hypochlorites in dirty wounds only,

Table 5.3 Summary of randomised, controlled trials of leg ulcer dressings (the numbers in the columns refer to the reference which relates to that trial)

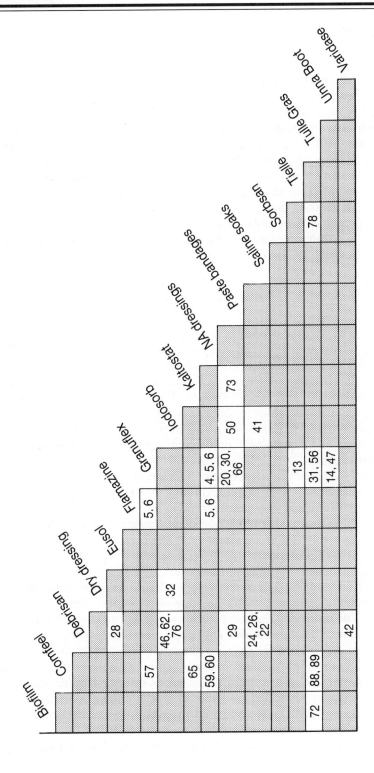

whilst Calder and Leaper themselves (1986) advocated the use of Eusol for debridement.

However, the lack of data demonstrating the beneficial effects of these products, matched against the wealth of data suggesting possible detrimental effects, would tend to petition against their use. Many of the modern wound dressings clean and debride wounds as successfully and with less risk. Thus while wound cleansing and debridement is indicated in certain circumstances, it is clear that we have insufficient evidence concerning when to cleanse, how to cleanse and when to stop. Current opinion favours regular washing of the ulcerated leg by immersing it in a bucket of warm water or by the patient soaking in an immersion bath or shower (Centre for Medical Education, University of Dundee, 1992). The ulcer may be cleansed at dressing time (if necessary) using warmed tap water or saline. Clinical infection, indicated by pain, inflammation, heat and purulent exudate should be treated by systemic antibiotics, as topical antibiotics are potent sensitizers (*British Medical Journal*, 1977).

Enzymic Debridement

A number of enzymic debriding agents are available, or are under development. A mixture of streptokinase and streptodornase (Varidase™, Lederle) is the most commonly used enzymic debriding agent in the UK. The streptokinase component converts inactive plasminogen to active plasmin, a proteolytic enzyme involved in the degradation of fibrin and fibrinogen. The streptodornase component comprises a group of enzymes which liquify deoxyribonucleoprotein, a large component of pus (Hellgren and Vincent, 1977). The preparation is recommended for use in the degradation and liquefaction of necrotic tissue, blood clots and fibrinous and purulent exudate.

In vitro studies of the effect of streptokinase-streptodornase on necrotic material harvested from leg ulcers, suggested that it breaks up fibrin and purulent exudate more successfully than the enzyme trypsin (Trypure), though the preparations were equipotent against 3 day old blood clots (Hellgren and Vincent, 1977). This *in vitro* study involved a crude visual estimate, rather than objective measurement, of the extent of proteolysis.

The relative clinical efficacies of streptokinase-streptodornase (Varidase) versus trypsin were examined in a randomized clinical trial involving 40 patients with vascular leg ulcers of differing aetiologies (Hellgren, 1983). The endpoint was complete debridement (judged by observers blind to the treatment used), rather than complete healing. Although streptokinase-streptodornase achieved more rapid debridement over 21 days, no difference between treatments with respect to extent of granulation, oedema and erythema was observed. Neither preparation was very effective against deep, hard necrosis or dry gangrene and the twice-daily dressing changes advocated are likely to preclude their use in the community.

Suomalainen (1983) also compared streptokinase-streptodornase and trypsin in 38 patients with traumatic ulcers, but again the effect of a period of debridement on time to complete healing of ulceration was not determined. Similar numbers in each group had begun to epithelialise during the 2 week study, though streptokin-ase-streptodornase was judged (using five point visual rating scales) to be the more effective debriding agent.

Forsling (1988) compared streptokinase-streptodornase with saline in a random-ised controlled trial involving 31 patients with 'oozing' leg ulcers. The endpoint of the trial was only 15 days, at which point the amount of pus and debris was evaluated by a 'blinded' observer. Ninety-two per cent of the wounds in the active treatment group were judged clean in 10 days compared with 50 per cent of the control group; however, the effect of the treatments on healing time was not evaluated.

Therefore there is evidence that enzymic preparations can speed up cleaning and debridement, but whether this affects the time to complete healing is unclear, though it may shorten preparation time prior to skin grafting. In addition, the properties of enzyme preparations are dependent on their careful use, since the protein components are denatured by exposure to heat or rough handling. Enzymic preparations are expensive and further research is required to determine whether cost-effective treatment regimens viable for community use are a possi-bility.

HYDROCOLLOID DRESSINGS

INDICATIONS: light to moderately exuding wounds; dry, necrotic wounds; granu-lating wounds.

The Evidence

A number of hydrocolloid dressings are now available in the UK, e.g. Biofilm™ (Clinimed), Comfeel™ (Coloplast), Granuflex™ (Convatec) and Tegasorb™ (3M). The relative compositions of these dressings vary (reviewed by Thomas, 1990), but they all contain colloids, elastomeric and adhesive components (Turner, 1986). Granuflex, the first hydrocolloid dressing to be introduced into the UK (1970s), is comprised of sodium carboxymethylcellulose, polyisobutylene, gelatin and pectin.

Some hydrocolloid dressings are available in a range of formulations, including granules, and sheets of differing thicknesses and performance profiles. Granuflex is available incorporated into a compression bandage system. Hydrocolloids are generally regarded as impermeable to gases including water vapour; however, Thomas's careful laboratory studies of dressings' performance have indicated that different hydrocolloids display a range of water vapour permeabilities, Granuflex being one of the more permeable (Thomas, 1990). Hydrocolloids tend to absorb wound exudate, forming a gel or paste. They are therefore interactive with the wound surface, and maintain a high level of humidity at the wound-dressing interface thus allowing moist wound healing. Most of the comparative trials of hydrocolloids undertaken thus far have investigated the performance of Granuflex, marketed as Duoderm™ in the US.

Laboratory studies using a chick model have demonstrated that Granuflex induces the growth of new blood vessels, to a greater extent than gauze (Amery et al, 1986), an equivalent weight of Silastic foam or no dressing (Cherry and Ryan, 1985). A study of full-thickness wounds in pigs demonstrated a significantly greater angiogenic effect in Granuflex than the semi-permeable film dressing, Opsite (Lydon et al, 1988). However, studies by Ulrek et al (1990a) using the same chick model found virtually no angiogenic effect associated with either Granuflex or Comfeel compared with angiogenic growth factor as a positive control. Thus it is probable that if occlusive dressings such as hydrocolloids stimulate new blood vessel growth, it is probably due to the low oxygen tension they produce rather than the presence of growth factors in the dressings.

Granuflex is also reported to demonstrate the ability to break down fibrin (Lydon et al, 1988), a potentially valuable property given the presence of fibrin cuffs and diminished fibrinolytic activity in ulcer patients; however, the clinical significance of this report was criticised by Ulrek et al (1990b) who reported that the natural catalyst fibrin is 1000 times more potent than either Granuflex or Comfeel.

The most rigorously controlled trials of Granuflex in wound healing are those of Backhouse et al (1987) and Blair et al (1988a, b) of the Department of Surgery at Charing Cross Hospital. Backhouse et al (1987) randomised 56 patients with chronic venous ulcers to receive either Granuflex or NA dressings underneath the Charing Cross four-layer bandage system. Life table analysis of the healing data demonstrated no significant difference between the two dressings, with 75 per cent healing at 12 weeks in the Granuflex group and 78 per cent in the NA dressing group. Blair et al (1988a) compared Granuflex, NA dressings and Flamazine (1 per cent silver sulphadiazine cream, Smith & Nephew) under the same four-layer bandage system in 120 patients and found no significant differences: 73 per cent healing at 12 weeks in Granuflex, 77 per cent in the NA dressing group and 63 per cent in the Flamazine group. These workers concluded that dressing choice is irrelevant; however, the applicability of these findings to the clinical situation is *severely* limited by the fact that ulcers with an area of more than 10 cm^2 were excluded. The mean ulcer size in the Backhouse et al study was only 3 cm^2. It is possible therefore that the trial focused on a late stage of the healing process when there was little likelihood of detecting a difference between dressings.

Granuflex has been compared with paste bandages in three controlled studies, the Unna boot in two studies, and tulle gras in two studies. Eriksson (1985b) compared zinc oxide paste plus Tensoplast bandage with Granuflex dressing plus compression in 34 patients with venous ulcers. No detail of the compression provided to the Granuflex group was given. Forty two per cent complete healing was reported in the paste bandage group compared with 53 per cent in the hydrocolloid group at 12 weeks. Groenewald (1985) also compared Granuflex with zinc oxide paste bandage, but a lack of information regarding the compression applied in each group makes evaluation of his findings difficult. No complete healing data was presented; however, there was a mean reduction in ulcer size of 22.6 per cent in the control group against 67.7 per cent in the hydrocolloid group.

Robinson (1988) randomized 133 patients with venous ulceration to receive either Viscopaste PB7 paste bandage or Granuflex hydrocolloid dressing. Both groups received identical compression systems, i.e. two layers of shaped tubular bandage (Tubigrip™, Seton). Unfortunately the study only lasted 8 weeks—too short a time to follow an appreciable proportion of patients to complete healing and no significant difference in healing rates between the groups was detected.

Kikta et al (1988) compared the Unna boot to Duoderm in patients with venous ulcers; however, they failed to provide those patients in the Duoderm group with any compression. Unfortunately as the Unna boot itself does provide compression, the wound contact material is not the only difference between the two groups and the fact that 64 per cent of ulcers in the Unna boot group were healed at 15 weeks compared with 35 per cent in the Duoderm is probably due to the lack of compression in the latter group. Cordts et al (1992) acknowledged the shortcomings of the Kikta study, and undertook a comparison of the Unna boot and Duoderm plus Coban compression bandage in patients with venous ulcers. No significant difference in healing rates was observed; however, the study was small (30 patients) and only 12 weeks in duration.

Handfield-Jones et al (1988) randomized hospital inpatients to either Granuflex or the tulle dressing Jelonet™ (Smith & Nephew); however, the design of the study (cross-over of treatment at only 3 weeks) and its small sample size (10 subjects) diminishes the usefulness of the findings (no difference in efficacy was detected). Meredith and Gray (1988) randomized 49 community patients to either Granuflex or Jelonet. All patients in this study received either Elastocrepe or straight Tubigrip, neither of which provide adequate compression. Seventy six per cent complete healing was reported in the Granuflex group at 6 weeks compared with 25 per cent in the Jelonet group; however, no patient-related data was presented and the comparability of groups on entry to the trial was not provided.

A couple of other studies have compared Duoderm/Granuflex to new dressings. Brandrup et al (1990) conducted a randomized trial of an occlusive zinc dressing (Mezinc, Molnlycke) and Duoderm in 43 patients with ulcers of various aetiologies. This trial was only short in duration, so only eight patients had healed completely in this time (four in each group). Collier (1992) compared Tielle™ (Johnson & Johnson), a new semi-permeable dressing comprising absorbent hydrophilic foam and Granuflex in patients with ulcers defined as venous or arterial. This trial lasted only 8 weeks and no detail of the compression provided to patients with venous insufficiency was given. Very little data was presented in this study, and therefore the claim that the Tielle dressing provides "significant advantages over hydrocolloids" must be viewed with scepticism.

Comfeel is another hydrocolloid dressing which like Granuflex contains sodium carboxymethylcellulose; however, it is different in both formulation and presentation (see Thomas, 1990). Comfeel has bevelled edges and becomes transparent when the dressing needs replacing. Winter and Cameron (1990) and Winter and Hewitt (1990) compared Comfeel and Jelonet in patients with either leg ulcers or pressure sores. It is unclear whether these reports constitute two separate studies, or two reports of the same study. Winter and Cameron studied 50 patients with 61 leg ulcers/pressure sores but their report is both scanty and descriptive. Winter and Hewitt (1990) in a similar study of 114 patients with 141 leg ulcers and pressure sores reported 63 per cent complete healing at 12 weeks in the Comfeel-treated group against 19 per cent in the Jelonet-treated group. No details of baseline comparability of the groups were presented, nor was there a breakdown of results in relation to wound type.

Rainey (1993) compared the performance of Comfeel Extra Absorbing Dressing™ (Coloplast) with the alginate Kaltostat™ (Britcair) in a small ($n = 19$) randomised controlled trial in patients with highly exuding leg ulcers. Unfortunately no healing data was reported for these patients and the data presented was purely descriptive with no statistical analysis; however, the author concluded that the Comfeel dressing had certain advantages over the alginate in terms of its water resistance, lack of strike-through, ease of removal and acceptability to nurses.

Although the team at Charing Cross are well known for their advocacy of simple non-adherent dressings (Backhouse et al, 1987; Blair et al, 1988a, b), a fascinating study by Moffatt et al (1992a, b) explored the use of Comfeel in cases of recalcitrant leg ulceration. Patients were included into this study if they had ulcers which had failed to heal within 24 weeks or failed to reduce in size by more than 20 per cent. This study of 60 patients was not confined to patients with small ulcers and those included ranged in size up to 66 cm². Comfeel did appear to confer an advantage in these patients, with 43 per cent achieving complete healing at 12 weeks in the Comfeel group compared with 23 per cent in the control group who received NA dressings. This difference did not quite reach significance at the $P < 0.05$ level, possibly because the sample size was not large enough to detect a difference.

Another type of hydrocolloid, Biofilm (Clinimed) has been compared to the local standard treatment of paraffin tulle (Jelonet, Smith & Nephew) and Betadine in a large randomised controlled trial involving 200 patients (Smith et al, 1992). Patients were stratified by ulcer size into those with ulcers of 2–4 cm diameter and those with larger ulcers. Compression was standardised and consisted of either two layers of shaped Tubigrip or Venosan 2002 compression stockings. Outcomes evaluated included pain and comfort as well as healing. Leg ulcers treated with Biofilm healed more rapidly, but not significantly so; however, patients receiving Biofilm experienced significantly less pain than those receiving Jelonet and Betadine.

There is little doubt that hydrocolloids provide a useful addition to the array of dressings available for managing leg ulcers; however, those studies undertaken so far have been small scale with little replication. The ability of hydrocolloids to reduce pain and allow the patient to bathe are certainly useful and their ability to contain relatively large volumes of exudata reduces the frequency of district nursing visits required if a patient is managed at home.

How does one choose *between* the different hydrocolloids available? Few studies have tackled this question and one is unlikely to demonstrate significant differences in healing rates between such similar products. Choice is much more likely to be determined by the 'handleability' of the different products, as well as other factors such as cost, smell, colour, shape and patient preference. Milward (1991) compared Granuflex and Comfeel in a randomized trial involving 50 patients, and collected data relating to nurse satisfaction, patient comfort and acceptability. This study reported a significant difference in the number of problems with leakage of exudate between the two dressings—more problems being encountered with Granuflex. The fact that the colour of Comfeel changes to become transparent when it requires changing was greatly appreciated by nurses, as was its bevelled edge which was felt to help the application of compression hosiery over the dressing.

In his review of 1986, Turner remarked that though the advent of hydrogels and hydrocolloids marked a new era in wound management, the fact that they are interactive dressings which release polysaccharides in a gel form at the wound interface requires examination. He wrote:

"The release of monomers subsequent to biodegradation is a possibility, and the interaction of these monomers with the biosystem should be considered."

In 1991, Young et al published an animal study, wherein dermal repair under Opsite film dressing and Granuflex hydrocolloid was examined at the cellular level. After 5 days, Granuflex-treated wounds demonstrated a granuloma-type reaction, possibly as a response to particles of foreign material. Examination of Granuflex-treated wounds after 160 days showed that the hypodermis of each wound contained cavities surrounded by inflammatory cells. However, the Granuflex dressings were left in contact with the wound for 21 days, a time period far in excess of the manufacturer's recommendations. The clinical and toxicological implications of these findings are unclear; whether this prolonged inflammatory reaction is due to the excessive time the dressing had been left in place, is peculiar to the pig model or is peculiar to Granuflex or all hydrocolloid dressings is not known. However, the finding should not be ignored. A long-term follow-up study of hydrocolloid-treated wounds (both experimental and clinical), possibly including the taking of biopsies, is advisable in the light of this report.

BEAD DRESSINGS

INDICATIONS: sloughy, dirty wounds.

The Evidence

There are two bead-type dressings marketed in the UK: cadexomer iodine (Iodosorb™, Perstorp Pharma) and dextranomer (Debrisan™, Pharmacia). Both are hydrophilic, polysaccharide bead preparations; the former containing iodine.

Dextranomer

Dextranomer, as Debrisan (Pharmacia) (beads 0.1–0.3 mm in diameter), is available in bead, paste and absorbent pad formulations. One gram of Debrisan is capable of absorbing up to 4 ml of fluid (Heel et al, 1979). Debrisan is advocated for moist, yellow, sloughy wounds (Thomas, 1990) and acts as a cleansing agent by virtue of its hydrophilic nature; drawing molecules with molecular weight less than 1000 into the beads, and larger molecules including wound debris and microorganisms into the matrix between the beads.

The effectiveness of Debrisan versus a number of other therapies for leg ulcer management has been examined in several randomised, controlled trials (table 5.4); however, interpretation of these findings can be problematic. There is no consensus as to the best method of quantifying cleansing and debridement, and the interpretation of studies is usually subjective, with the likelihood of observer bias. The question of whether using these materials for a short time to clean up a sloughy wound actually reduces time to complete healing has not been answered. Only one small study has examined the effect of Debrisan use on total healing time (Kero et al, 1987), and although studies report that Debrisan has good cleansing and debriding effects most studies are too small or short in duration to demonstrate a benefit in terms of reducing healing time.

Marzin (1993) compared Debrisan absorbent pads with the Debrisan Paste in 80 patients with venous leg ulcers in a randomised controlled trial. Since Debrisan Pads are essentially Debrisan Paste in a polyamide bag it would have been very surprising if this study demonstrated any difference in healing rates (it did not). The presence of pus, debris, pain, necrotic tissue, granulation tissue and epithelialisation was assessed (no detail of how this was done is given) and ulcer area was measured. No difference between the products in any aspect of performance was observed, however the author concluded that the pads were easier to use.

Cadexomer Iodine

Cadexomer iodine (Iodosorb, Perstorp Pharma) consists of hydrophilic beads containing 0.9 per cent w/w iodine. The uptake of aqueous media into the beads (1 g Idosorb absorbs up to 7 ml fluid) results in liberation of the iodine. Iodosorb is also available as both beads and paste, and again is indicated for moist, sloughy exuding wounds (Thomas, 1990). Its use is contraindicated in patients with known iodine sensitivity.

Randomised, controlled clinical trials of Iodosorb in leg ulcers are summarised in table 5.5. Although Iodosorb appears to contribute to ulcer cleaning, the poor quality of trials thus far does not provide evidence for Iodosorb decreasing the time to complete healing for leg ulcers.

PASTE BANDAGES AND UNNA BOOTS

INDICATIONS: venous ulcers generally, and particularly those where eczema is present.

Table 5.4 Summary of randomised, controlled clinical trials of Debrisan as a leg ulcer therapy

Reference	Comparison	Reported outcome	Comments
Floden and Wikstrom (1978)	Debrisan versus saline soaks in venous ulcers (51 patients)	Debrisan better at promoting granulation, clearing pus and debris, reducing pain	Compression not standardised; effect on complete healing unreported; assessment scales of questionable validity
Frank et al (1979)	Debrisan versus saline soaks in venous ulcers (20 patients)	Subjective analysis only	Beads associated with burning sensation and difficulty with removal
Groenewald (1980)	Effect of including Debrisan in standard treatment of povidone iodine, Eusol, zinc oxide paste, compression (100 patients)	96% Debrisan ulcers cleaned in mean 5.9 days cf. 60% in 15.4 days in controls	Effect on healing time unreported.
Groenewald (1981)	Debrisan versus paste bandage and compression (100 patients)	Debrisan cleaned ulcers more quickly	No compression in Debrisan group; no patient/ulcer details presented; effect on healing time unreported.
Sawyer et al (1978, 1979)	Standard debridement (mechanical, chlorhexidine or betadine) with or without Debrisan (60 patients)	More complete healing in Debrisan group but time period not clear	Ulcers of varying aetiology; criteria for 'healing' or 'failure' unclear; optional cross-over at 3 weeks.
Hulkko et al (1981)	Debrisan versus Varidase (28 patients)	Both agents said to be good cleansers; more granulation tissue with Debrisan	Only subjective assessment of effectiveness; effect on complete healing unreported.
Kero et al (1987)	Debrisan versus Iodosorb (27 patients)	50% healing in 8 weeks in Debrisan group cf. 65% in Iodosorb group	
Moss et al (1987)	Debrisan versus Iodosorb (42 patients)	No difference between groups reported (as % change in area of ulcers)	Complicated by optional cross-over at 6 weeks; no detail of compression therapy.
Eriksson et al (1984)	Debrisan versus saline soaks (53 patients)	No difference between groups for healing	This comparative study lasted only two weeks at the commencement of a trial of three other treatments.
Marzin (1993)	Debrisan Pads versus Debrisan Paste (n = 80)	No significant difference with respect to any of the parameters measured.	Treatment was renewed daily or twice daily. No detail of compression. No detail of how pus, debris, necrosis, pain, granulation, epithelialisation actually assessed.
Tarvainen (1988)	Debrisan versus Iodosorb (27 patients)	No difference reported between groups	Only 8 weeks study so no complete healing data; eight of 27 patients withdrew

Table 5.5   Summary of randomised, controlled clinical trials of Iodosorb as a leg ulcer therapy

Reference	Comparison	Reported outcome	Comments
Harcup and Saul (1986)	Iodosorb versus dry dressing +/− antiseptics including Eusol (72 patients)	Greater reduction in mean ulcer size, oedema, erythema, exudate, odour, pus, pain at 4 weeks in Iodosorb group	Ulcers in Iodosorb group smaller at baseline; optional cross-over at 4 weeks; randomisation not adhered to; no complete healing data
Hillstrom (1988)	Iodosorb versus various 'standard' treatments (74 patients)	Greater % reduction in area in Iodosorb group; more granulation; less puss and debris	Demonstrates ineffectiveness of standard therapy rather than effectiveness of Iodosorb
Ormiston et al (1985)	Iodosorb versus standard therapy of gentian violet and topical antibiotics (61 patients)	40% healing at 12 weeks in Iodosorb group cf. 23% in control group	Poor healing in both groups; patients largely self-caring
Skog et al (1983)	Iodosorb versus antiseptic cleansing and non-adherent dressings (93 patients)	Greater reduction in mean ulcer size in Iodosorb group; also less pus, debris, exudate, more granulation	No detail of compression; no complete healing data; question clinical significance of slight differences between groups; validity of wound assessment scales not demonstrated
Steele et al (1986)	Iodosorb versus standard therapy of topical antibiotics, antiseptics, steroids (114 patients)	No reported difference re: ulcer size, pus, debris, granulation	Control therapy likely to inhibit healing; no complete healing data; no proper compression; control therapy varied.
Holloway et al (1989)	Iodosorb versus saline soaks (75 patients)	Greater reported rate of healing in Iodosorb group (expressed as cm² per week but ulcers not of comparable initial size)	Ulcers initially larger in Iodosorb group and larger ulcers heal at an initially faster rate; no complete healing data; no detail of compression.
Laudanska and Gustavson (1988)	Iodosorb versus paste bandage (67 patients)	Greater % reduction in ulcer area in Iodosorb group at 6 weeks	No complete healing data; patients in hospital on bed rest; three patients excluded from analysis as ulcers too big to measure (but does not say which group they were in)
Moss et al (1987) Kero et al (1987) Tarvainen (1988)	Iodosorb versus Debrisan Iodosorb versus Debrisan Iodosorb versus Debrisan		See table 5.4

The Evidence

The paste bandage is one of the most widely-used leg ulcer dressings in the UK and exists in a number of formulations. Paste bandages consist of plain weave cotton fabric impregnated with zinc oxide paste either alone (Zincaband™, Seton; Viscopaste PB7™ (Smith & Nephew); or with calamine (Calaband™, Seton); calamine and clioquinol (Quinaband™, Seton); coal tar (Coltapaste™, Smith & Nephew; Tarband™, Seton); or icthammol (Icthopaste™, Smith & Nephew; Icthoband™, Seton). These additives are proposed to soothe the eczema so commonly associated with venous ulceration. Paste bandages are applied fairly loosely from toe to knee, taking care to avoid a tourniquet effect either by doubling the bandage back on itself or cutting and applying in strips to avoid encircling the leg. It is necessary to apply a secondary bandage over the paste bandage to preserve its moisture, and in the case of patients with venous insufficiency, to apply compression.

Surprisingly, despite the popularity of the paste bandage system, few published studies have compared its effectiveness to other leg ulcer systems. Eriksson (1985b, 1986) compared the efficacy of zinc oxide paste bandage plus Tensoplast compression bandage with Granuflex dressing plus Wero elastic bandage. The subbandage pressure delivered by each system was not measured. Seven out of 17 ulcers treated with paste plus Tensoplast healed in 12 weeks, compared with nine out of 17 treated wwith Granuflex plus Wero elastic bandage, but the sample size was too small to be certain that important differences between the two systems would be detected. It is worth noting that the Granuflex system required changing up to twice a week compared with the paste system which required a weekly or fortnightly change.

Travers et al (1991a, b) compared the outcomes in 15 patients treated with a new self-adhesive, short-stretch bandage, Panelast acryl™, to eight patients treated with a three-layer system of Calaband (Seton) paste bandage, Tensopress™ and Tensogrip™ (Smith & Nephew). Panelast acryl delivered a mean pressure of 49 mmHg falling to 22 mmHg over a week, compared with 44.5 mmHg falling to 36.2 mmHg over a week in the three-layer system. No difference was reported in the healing rates produced by the two systems, although the small number of patients in the study increases the likelihood of missing a real difference even if there was one. Importantly, the one-layer system is less time-consuming to apply.

The study by Robinson (1988) described earlier found no difference in healing rates in ulcers treated with either Viscopaste PB7 paste bandage or Granuflex hydrocolloid dressing; however, the clinical significance of this finding cannot be ascertained as the study was only 8 weeks in duration.

Finally, Stacey et al (1992) conducted a randomised controlled trial involving 113 patients with venous ulcers to receive either Viscopaste PB7 paste bandage, Kaltostat (an alginate dressing) or Acoband (zinc oxide in stockingette form). The three groups received an identical compression system in the form of two Elastocrepe bandages and a layer of Tubigrip. Patients receiving the Viscopaste fared significantly better than the patients receiving Acoband or Kaltostat. Sixty six per cent of patients receiving Viscopaste were completely healed at 3 months, compared with 50 per cent of the Acoband group and 45 per cent of the group which received Kaltostat.

Thus, the results of three out of the four published randomised controlled trials of paste bandages are difficult to interpret due to either the small numbers of patients involved (Eriksson, 1985b, 1986; Travers et al, 1991a, b) or the short duration of the study (Robinson, 1988). The only study which followed a large sample of patients to complete healing demonstrated Viscopaste to have an advantage over Kaltostat or Acoband. This advantage may be due to the provision of extra compression during walking applied by the paste bandage.

Unfortunately, perservatives contained in paste bandages produce contact sensitivity in a proportion of susceptible individuals (see chapter 9 for a full discussion of this problem).

The Unna boot

The Unna boot is a non-compliant plaster-type dressing dating from the 1850s and little used in the UK, though widely used elsewhere including the US. Unna Boots are similar to the paste bandages so widely used in the UK, except they contain glycerine and harden to a semi-rigid boot thus providing compression as well as a wound dressing.

The efficacy of Unna boots has been examined in five randomised, controlled trials of venous ulcer healing. However, four out of the five studies were confounded and their value reduced by the existence of substantial differences in the care of the patients in the two treatment groups (Hendricks and Swallow, 1985); a lack of detail of the compression provided or a lack of any compression given to the control group (Sikes, 1985; Kikta et al, 1988). The best evaluation of the Unna boot compared Duoderm (Granuflex in the UK) plus Coban compression bandage to Unna's boot in a 12 week study (Cordts et al, 1992). Fifty per cent of patients in the Duoderm group compared with 43 per cent in the Unna boot group were completely healed at 12 weeks. This was a small study of 30 patients and this may be the reason why no significant difference was found between the groups.

ALGINATE DRESSINGS

INDICATIONS: exuding wounds.

The Evidence

Alginate dressings have been developed from seaweed derivatives and contain calcium alginate (e.g. Sorbsan™, Steriseal), or a mixture of calcium and sodium alginates in the case of Kaltostat (BritCair). Both products are available as flat dressing pads or in rope forms for packing cavity wounds, and require cover by a secondary dressing. When the alginate material comes into contact with wound exudate or serum, sodium ions in the body fluid are exchanged with the calcium ions in the dressing, forming a more soluble sodium alginate. The dressing becomes a hydrophilic gel which creates a moist healing environment at the wound interface. This gel can be irrigated from the wound using saline at dressing changes. The high absorptive capacity of the alginates makes them ideal dressings for highly exuding wounds, and their use should be avoided in dry or lightly exuding wounds as they may dry the wound bed, and be difficult to remove.

Thomas (1989) carried out a randomized controlled trial of Sorbsan on 64 leg ulcers. Paraffin tulle was used as a control. Only one ulcer in the control group healed, compared with 31 per cent of ulcers in the Sorbsan group; however, the time taken to complete healing was not reported, and the value of these findings is diminished as compression was not standardized and many patients received no compression at all. Ulcers in the control group were of longer duration and very little baseline information about the patients was presented. The trial by Stacey et al (1992) described above reported 20 per cent more ulcer healing under Viscopaste PB7 paste bandage than Kaltostat. Rainey (1993) compared Kaltostat with Comfeel Extra Absorbing Dressing (also described above); however, this study did not report healing rates. Moffatt et al (1992c) evaluated the calcium alginate dressing Tegagel™ (3M) in a randomized controlled trial involving 60 patients, using NA dressing (Johnson & Johnson) as the control. Only patients with small ulcers (area less than 3 cm^2) were included in this study and all patients received the standard four-layer, high compression bandage. No significant difference in healing rates was observed and healing rates were very high in both groups (87 per cent complete healing at 12 weeks in the Tegagel group compared with 80 per cent in the NA dressing group).

A number of other dressings are commonly used in the management of leg ulcers, for which there is a relative or absolute lack of published research regarding their effectiveness. One published study has evaluated the effectiveness of Allevyn™ (Smith & Nephew), a hydrocellular polyurethane dressing capable of absorbing large volumes of exudate (Callam et al, 1992). The patients in the control group in this randomised trial received the low-adherent dressing Tricotex™ (Smith & Nephew). The ulcers in this study appear to have been fairly small as the mean ulcer size in the Allevyn group was 8.35 and 10.87 cm^2 in the Tricotex group. At the end of 12 weeks, 47 per cent of ulcers in the Allevyn group compared with 35 per cent in the Tricotex group were completely healed; however, the difference did not reach significance at the $P<0.5$ level.

Other products available but under-researched include the hydrogel Intrasite Gel™ (Smith & Nephew), which rehydrates sloughy, necrotic wounds and promotes autolysis of devitalised tissue (the body's own debridement mechanism) and foam dressings such as Lyofoam™ (Seton) which are indicated for heavily exuding wounds. Information regarding the use of these and other dressings can be found in Thomas's *A Handbook of Surgical Dressings* (1992).

Skin grafting may also be used to speed up healing and cover epithelial defects. A variety of skin grafting techniques exist; a piece of skin may be taken from a donor site such as the thigh and applied intact, or skin may be meshed or shredded to give expansion. Grafts may be autologous (removed from the patient himself) or allografts (from donors), and may be grown in cell culture. A randomised controlled trial of pinch skin grafting demonstrated beneficial effects; however, the control group in this study received porcine skin as a dressing (Poskitt et al, 1987) and it is perhaps not too surprising that an autologous skin graft proved more effective. It is unclear to what extent skin grafting is used in the treatment of leg ulcer patients, and largely speaking this is an area of medical responsibility although the taking and application of pinch skin grafts is viewed as part of the role of the nurse in certain areas (Moffatt and Oldroyd, 1989).

SUMMARY

- This chapter has summarized the evidence from randomised controlled trials of topical leg ulcer products (Table 5.3). The research evidence provides little in the way of direction for those making clinical decisions, however the number and rigour of trials appears to be increasing.
- Fundamental research is required to examine what makes a chronic wound 'chronic'.
- There is good evidence that a moist environment is the optimum for wound healing. Modern dressings such as the hydrocolloids, hydrogels and semipermeable films provide such an environment. There is no evidence of increased infection rates under occlusive dressings.
- Low oxygen tension appears to stimulate wound healing.
- Most ulcers are colonized by microorganisms but there is little evidence to suggest they affect ulcer healing. The effect of systemic antibiotics or topical antiseptics on time to complete healing has not been measured.
- Clinical infection of leg ulcers should be treated with systemic antibiotics.
- Animal studies suggest that the presence of devitalised tissue in a wound decreases the ability of leucocytes to ingest bacteria.
- No clinical trial has examined the role of cleansing and debridement in total healing times. The use of enzymic debriding agents appears to facilitate ulcer cleansing, but no study has measured the effect of the use of such agents (for a period) on total healing time.
- The lack of data demonstrating the beneficial effects of hypochlorites, coupled with evidence from animal and *in vitro* studies of harmful effects, persuades against their use. Expert opinion favours bathing the leg in warm tap water or cleansing with saline.
- More research is required into the best means and appropriate time to cleanse ulcers.
- Trials of dressings are often confounded by a lack of standardisation of compression therapy and include too small a sample size to detect any difference between two products (if one exists). Many trials are of too short a duration to follow sufficent ulcers to complete healing.
- Bead-type dressings appear to facilitate cleansing and desloughing; however, only two trials have examined the effect of their use on complete healing.

Both studies used small sample sizes and the contribution of these agents is not clear.

● The taking and application of pinch skin grafts is seen as part of the extended role of the nurse in some areas; however, the only randomized, controlled clinical trial of pinch skin grafting compared the practice with the effectiveness of porcine skin as a dressing.

References

Alvarez O M, Mertz P M and Eaglstein W H (1983) The effect of occlusive dressings on collagen synthesis and re-epithelialization in superficial wounds. *Journal of Surgical Research*, **35**: 142–148.

Amery M J, Ryan T J and Cherry G W (1986) Successful treatment of venous ulcers with a new hydrocolloid dressing—passive or active in wound healing. In: *Phlebology '85*, eds Negus D and Jantet G, London: Libbey.

Backhouse C M, Blair S D, Savage A P, Walton J and McCollum C N (1987) Controlled trial of occlusive dressings in healing chronic venous ulcers. *British Journal of Surgery*, **74**: 626–627.

Blair S D, Backhouse C M, Wright D D I, Riddle E and McCollum C N (1988a) Do dressings influence the healing of chronic venous ulcers? *Phlebology*, **3**: 129–134.

Blair S D, Wright D D, Backhouse C M, Riddle E and McCollum C N (1988b) Sustained compression and healing of chronic venous ulcers. *British Medical Journal*, **297**: 1159–1161.

Brandrup F, Menne T, Agren M S, Stromberg H E, Holst R and Frisen M (1990) A randomized trial of two occlusive dressings in the treatment of leg ulcers. *Acta Dermatologia Venereologia Stockholm*, **70**: 231–235.

Brennan S S and Leaper D J (1985) The effect of antiseptics on the healing wound: a study using the rabbit ear chamber. *British Journal of Surgery*, **72**: 780–782.

British Medical Journal (1977) Topical antibiotics. *British Medical Journal*, **1**: 1494.

Calder S J and Leaper D J (1986) Chronic venous leg ulcers and the role of dressings in their treatment. *Bristol Medico-Chirurgical Journal*, **101**: 6–9, 11.

Callam M J, Harper D R, Dale J J, Brown D and Gibson B (1992) Lothian and Forth Valley Leg Ulcer Healing Trial Part 2: knitted viscose dressing versus a hydrocellular dressing in the treatment of chronic leg ulceration. *Phlebology*, **7**: 142–145.

Centre for Medical Education, The University of Dundee (1992) *The Wound Programme*. Dundee: Centre for Medical Education, University of Dundee.

Cherry G W and Ryan T J (1985) Enhanced wound angiogenesis with a new hydrocolloid dressing. *Royal Society of Medicine International Congress & Symposium Series*, **85**: 61–68.

Collier J (1992) A moist, odour-free environment: a multicentre trial of a foamed gel and a hydrocolloid dressing. *Professional Nurse*, **7**: 804–808.

Cordts P R, Hanrahan L M, Rodriguez A A, Woodson J, LaMorte W W and Menzoian J O (1992) A prospective randomized trial of Unna's boot versus Duoderm CGF hydroactive dressing plus compression in the management of venous leg ulcers. *Journal of Vascular Surgery*, **15**: 480–486.

Cunliffe W J (1990) Eusol—to use or not to use? *Dermatology in Practice*, **April/May**: 5–6.

Dale J J (1986) Leg ulcers: treatments on trial. *Community Outlook*, **8**: 32–37.

Department of Health (1989) *A Strategy for Nursing: Report of the Steering Committee*. London: Department of Health.

Dyson M, Young S, Pendle C L, Webster D F and Land S M (1988) Comparison of the effects of moist and dry conditions on dermal repair. *Journal of Investigative Dermatology*, **91**: 434–439.

Eriksson G (1985a) Bacterial growth in venous leg ulcers—its clinical significance. *Royal Society of Medicine International Congress & Symposium Series*, **88**: 45–49.

Eriksson G (1985b) Comparative study of hydrocolloid dressing and double layer bandage in treatment of venous stasis ulceration. *Royal Society of Medicine International Congress & Symposium Series*, **88**: 111–121.

Eriksson G (1986) Comparison of two occlusive bandages in the treatment of venous leg ulcers. *British Journal of Dermatology*, **114**: 227–230.

Eriksson G, Eklund A E and Kallings L O (1984) The clinical significance of bacterial growth in venous leg ulcers. *Scandinavian Journal of Infectious Diseases*, **16**: 175–180.

Fletcher A (1992) Common problems of wound management in the elderly. In: *Proceedings of the 1st European Conference on Advances in Wound Management*. London: Macmillan Magazines.

Floden C-H and Wikstrom K (1978) Controlled clinical trial with dextranomer on venous leg ulcers. *Current Therapeutic Research*, **24**: 753–760.

Forsling E (1988) Comparison of saline and streptokinase-streptodornase in the treatment of leg ulcers. *European Journal of Clinical Pharmacology*, **33**: 637–638.

Frank D H, Robson M C and Heggers J P (1979) Evaluation of Debrisan as a treatment for leg ulcers. *Annals of Plastic Surgery*, **3**: 395–400.

Gilchrist B and Reed C (1989) The bacteriology of chronic venous ulcers treated with occlusive hydrocolloid dressings. *British Journal of Dermatology*, **121**: 337–344.

Groenewald J H (1980) An evaluation of dextranomer as a cleansing agent in the treatment of the post-phlebitic stasis ulcer. *South African Medical Journal*, **57**: 809–815.

Groenewald J H (1981) The treatment of varicose stasis ulcers: a controlled trial. *Schweiz Rundsch Med Praxis*, **70**: 1273–1278.

Groenewald J H (1985) Comparative effects of HCD and conventional treatment on the healing of venous stasis ulcers. *Royal Society of Medicine International Congress & Symposium Series*, **88**: 105–109.

Handfield-Jones S E, Grattan C E, Simpson R A and Kennedy C T (1988) Comparison of a hydrocolloid dressing and paraffin gauze in the treatment of venous ulcers. *British Journal of Dermatology*, **118**: 425–427.

Harcup J W, Saul P A (1986) A study of the effect of cadexomer iodine in the treatment of venous leg ulcers. *British Journal of Clinical Practice*, **40**: 360–364.

Haury B, Rodeheaver G, Vensko J, Edgerton M T and Edlich R F (1980) Debridement: An essential component of traumatic wound care. In: *Wound Healing and Wound Infection: Theory and Surgical Practice*, ed. Hunt T K, pp. 229–241. New York: Appleton-Century-Crofts.

Heel R C, Morton P, Brogden R N, Speight T M and Avery G S (1979) Dextranomer: a review of its general properties and therapeutic efficacy. *Drugs*, **18**: 89–102.

Hellgren L (1983) Cleansing properties of stabilized trypsin and streptokinase-streptodornase in necrotic leg ulcers. *European Journal of Clinical Pharmacology*, **24**: 623–628.

Hellgren L and Vincent J (1977) Degradation and liquefaction effect of streptokinase-streptodornase and stabilized trypsin on necroses, crusts of fibrinoid, purulent exudate and clotted blood from leg ulcers. *Journal of International Medical Research*, **5**, 334–337.

Hendricks W M and Swallow R T (1985) Management of stasis leg ulcers with Unna's boots versus elastic support stockings. *Journal of the American Academy of Dermatology*, **12**: 90–98.

Hillstrom L (1988) Iodosorb compared to standard treatment in chronic venous leg ulcers—a multicenter study. *Acta Chirurgica Scandinavica Supplementum*, **544**: 53–56.

Hinman C D and Maibach H (1963) Effect of air exposure and occlusion on experimental human skin wounds. *Nature*, **200**: 377–378.

Hohn D C, Ponce B, Burton R W and Hunt T K (1977) Antimicrobial systems of the surgical wound. *American Journal of Surgery*, **133**: 597–603.

Holloway G A Jr, Johansen K H, Barnes R W and Pierce G E (1989) Multicenter trial of cadexomer iodine to treat venous stasis ulcer. *Western Journal of Medicine*, **151**: 35–38.

Hulkko A, Holopainen Y V, Orava S, Kangas J, Kuusisto P, Hyvarinen E, Ervasti E and Silvennoinen E (1981) Comparison of dextranomer and streptokinase-streptodornase in the treatment of venous leg ulcers and other infected wounds. *Annales Chirurgiae et Gynaecologiae*, **70**: 65–70.

Hunt T K, Zederfeldt B and Goldstick T K (1969) Oxygen and healing. *American Journal of Surgery*, **118**: 521–525.

Hutchinson J J (1990) The rate of clinical infection in occluded wounds. In: *International Forum on Wound Microbiology*, eds Alexander J W, Thomson P D and Hutchinson J J, pp. 27–34. Princeton: Excerpta Medica.

Hutchinson J J (1992) Influence of occlusive dressings on wound microbiology: interim results of a multicentre clinical trial of an occlusive hydrocolloid dressing. In: *Proceedings of the 1st European Conference on Advances in Wound Management*, eds Harding K G, Leaper D L and Turner T D, pp. 152–155. London: Macmillan Magazines.

Kero M, Tarvainen K, Hollmen A and Pekanmaki K (1987) A comparison of cadexomer iodine with dextranomer in the treatment of venous leg ulcers. *Current Therapeutic Research*, **42**: 761–767.

Kikta M J, Schuler J J, Meyer J P, Durham J R, Eldrup-Jorgensen J, Schwarcz T H and Flanigan D P (1988) A prospective, randomized trial of Unna's boots versus hydroactive dressing in the treatment of venous stasis ulcers. *Journal of Vascular Surgery*, **7**: 478–483.

Knighton D R, Silver I A and Hunt T K (1981) Regulation of wound-healing angiogenesis-effect of oxygen gradients and inspired oxygen concentration. *Surgery*, **90**: 262–270.

Kozol R A, Gillies C and Elgebaly S A (1988) Effects of sodium hypochlorite (Dakin's Soln.) on cells of wound module. *Archives of Surgery*, **123**: 420–423.

Laudanska H and Gustavson B (1988) In-patient treatment of chronic varicose venous ulcers. A randomized trial of cadexomer iodine versus standard dressings. *Journal of International Medical Research*, **16**: 428–435.

Leaper D J and Brennan S S (1986) Lets have a rethink about the use of antiseptics for venous ulcers. In *Phlebology '85*, ed. Negus D and Jantet G. London: Libbey.

Lineaweaver W, Howard R, Soucy D, McMorris S, Freeman J, Crain C, Robertson J and Rumley T (1985) Topical antimicrobial toxicity. *Archives of Surgery*, **120**: 267–270.

Lydon M J, Cherry G W, Cederholm-Williams S A, Pickworth J J, Cherry C, Scudder G W, Johnson E R and Ryan T J (1988) Fibrinolytic activity of hydrocolloid dressing. *Royal Society of Medicine International Congress & Symposium Series*, **136**: 9–17.

Marzin L (1993) Comparing dextranomer absorbent pads and dextranomer paste in the treatment of venous leg ulcers. *Journal of Wound Care* **2**(2): 80–83.

McIntosh J B (1979) Decision-making on the district. *Nursing Times*, **75**(19): 77–80.

Meredith K and Gray E (1988) Dressed to heal. *Journal of District Nursing*, **7**(3): 8, 10.

Milward P (1991) Examining hydrocolloids. *Nursing Times*, **87**(36): 70–74.

Moffatt C and Oldroyd M (1989) Pinch skin grafting: an extension of the role of the clinical nurse specialist. *Primary Health Care*, **July**: 18–20.

Moffatt C J, Franks P J, Oldroyd M and Greenhalgh R M (1992a) Randomized trial of an occlusive dressing in the treatment of chronic non-healing leg ulcers. *Phlebology*, **7**: 105–107.

Moffatt C J, Oldroyd M I and Dickson D (1992b) A trial of a hydrocolloid dressing in the management of indolent ulceration. *Journal of Wound Care*, **1**(3): 20–22.

Moffatt C J, Oldroyd M I and Franks P J (1992c) Assessing a calcium alginate dressing for venous ulcers of the leg. *Journal of Wound Care*, **1**(4): 22–24.

Moss C, Taylor A E and Shuster S (1987) Comparison of cadexomer iodine and dextranomer for chronic venous ulcers. *Clinical and Experimental Dermatology*, **12**: 413–418.

Ormiston M C, Seymour M T, Venn G E, Cohen R I and Fox J A (1985) Controlled trial of Iodosorb in chronic venous ulcers. *British Medical Journal*, **291**: 308–310.

Poskitt K R, James A H, Lloyd-Davies E R, Walton J and McCollum C (1987) Pinch skin grafting or porcine dermis in venous ulcers: a randomised clinical trial. *British Medical Journal*, **294**: 674–676.

Rainey J (1993) A comparison of two dressings in the treatment of heavily exuding leg ulcers. *Journal of Wound Care*, **2**(4): 199–200.

Robinson B J (1988) Randomized comparative trial of Duoderm v's Viscopaste PB7 bandage in the management of venous leg ulceration and cost to the community. *Royal Society of Medicine International Congress & Symposium Series*, **136**: 101–104.

Sackett D L, Haynes R B, Guyatt G H and Tugwell P (1991) *Clinical Epidemiology: A Basic Science for Clinical Medicine*. Boston: Little Brown.

Sawyer P N, Sophie M D, Dowbak M D, Cohen M D and Feller J (1978) New approaches in the therapy of the peripheral vascular ulcer. *Angiology*, **29**: 666–674.

Sawyer P N, Dowbak G, Sophie Z, Feller J and Cohen L (1979) A preliminary report of the efficacy of Debrisan (dextranomer) in the debridement of cutaneous ulcers. *Surgery*, **85**: 201–204.

Sikes E (1985) Evaluation of a transparent dressing in the treatment of stasis ulcers of the lower limb. *Journal of Enterostomal Therapy*, **12**: 116–120.

Skog E, Arnesjo B, Troeng T, Gjores J E, Bergljung L, Gundersen J, Hallbook T, Hessman Y, Hillstrom L and Mansson T (1983) A randomized trial comparing cadexomer iodine and standard treatment in the out-patient management of chronic venous ulcers. *British Journal of Dermatology*, **109**: 77–83.

Smith J M, Doré C J, Charlett A and Lewis J D (1992) A randomized trial of Biofilm dressing for venous leg ulcers. *Phlebology*, **7**: 108–113.

Stacey M C, Jopp-McKay A G, Rashid P, Hoskin S E, Thompson P M (1992) The influence of dressings on venous ulcer healing. In: *Proceedings of the 1st European Conference on Advances in Wound Management*, eds Harding K G, Leaper D L, Turner T D, pp. 145–147. London: Macmillan Magazines.

Steele K, Irwin G, Dowds N (1986) Cadexomer iodine in the management of venous leg ulcers in general practice. *Practitioner*, **230**: 63–68.

Suomalainen O (1983) Evaluation of two enzyme preparations – trypure and varidase in traumatic ulcers. *Annales Chirurgiae et Gynaecologiae*, **72**: 62–65.

Tarvainen K (1988) Cadexomer iodine (Iodosorb) compared with dextranomer (Debrisan) in the treatment of chronic leg ulcers. *Acta Chirurgica Scandinavica Supplementum*, **544**: 57–59.

Tatnall F M, Leigh I M and Gibson J R (1987) Comparative toxicity of antimicrobial agents on transformed human keratinocytes. *Journal of Investigative Dermatology*, **89**: 316–317.

Thomas S (1989) Sorbsan in the management of leg ulcers. *Pharmaceutical Journal*, **243**: 706–709.

Thomas S (1990) *Wound Management and Dressings*. London: Pharmaceutical Press.

Thomas S (1992) *A Handbook of Surgical Dressings*, 1992 edn. Bridgend: Surgical Materials Testing Laboratory.

Tingle J (1990) Eusol and the law. *Nursing Times*, **86**(38): 70–72.

Travers J P, Dalziel K L, Makin G S (1991a) Assessment of a new, 1-layer self-adhesive bandage in sustained limb compression and venous ulcer healing. In: *Royal Society of Medicine Venous Forum Meeting*, London. October 25.

Travers J P, Dalziel K, Makin G S (1991b) Compression bandaging and venous ulcer healing: assessment of a new one layer bandaging technique. In: *2nd Joint British-Swedish Angiology Meeting*, London. September 11–13.

Turner T D (1986) Hydrogels and hydrocolloids—an overview of the products and their properties. In: *Advances in Wound Management*, ed. Turner T D, Schmidt R J and Harding K G, pp. 89–95. Chichester: John Wiley.

Ulrek D, Wilhelmsen F, Samuelsen P and Munk-Madsen S (1990a) Angiogenetic effect of hyrocolloid dressings. *Proceedings of the Conference: Clinical dermatology in the Year 2000*, May 22, London.

Ulrek D, Wilhelmsen F, Samuelsen P and Munk-Madsen S (1990b) Fibrinolysis and hydrocolloid dressings. *Proceedings of the Conference: Clinical dermatology in the Year 2000*, May 22, London.

Varghese M C, Balin A K, Carter D M and Caldwell D (1986) Local environment of chronic wounds under synthetic dressings. *Archives of Dermatology*, **122**: 52–57.

Winter A and Cameron S (1990) Healing in comfort. *Journal of District Nursing*, **July**.

Winter A and Hewitt H (1990) Testing a hydrocolloid. *Nursing Times*, **86**(50): 59–62.

Winter G D (1962) Formation of the scab and the rate of epithelialisation of superficial wounds in the skin of the young domestic pig. *Nature*, **193**: 293–294.

Young S R, Dyson M, Hickman R, Lang S and Osborn C (1991) Comparison of the effects of semi-occlusive polyurethane dressings and hydrocolloid dressings on dermal repair. 1. Cellular changes. *Journal of Investigative Dermatology*, **97**: 586–592.

6

Bandages used in Leg Ulcer

Management

INTRODUCTION

Although most experts agree that the application of graduated external compression is the single most important factor in the treatment of venous leg ulcers, there is rather less agreement concerning the degree of pressure required and the way in which this pressure should be achieved. This chapter is intended to provide an introduction to the role of compression, and to discuss those factors which determine the ability of a bandage or bandaging system to produce *and maintain* therapeutically effective levels of sub-bandage pressure.

THE ROLE OF COMPRESSION

As described in chapter 1, the veins of the leg are divided into the superficial and deep systems, linked together by vessels called perforators which contain valves that permit the flow of blood in one direction only; from the outer or superficial system inwards to the deep veins.

The venous pressure at the ankle in a subject who is lying supine is approximately 10 mmHg, but on standing this pressure will rise by about 80 mmHg, due to an increase in hydrostatic pressure (equivalent to the weight of a vertical column of blood stretching from the point of measurement to the right auricle of the heart).

During walking, as the foot is dorsal flexed, the contraction of the calf muscle compresses the deep veins to the point at which they become almost totally collapsed, producing internal pressures of up to 250 mmHg and emptying them of blood. As the foot is plantar flexed, the pressure in the veins falls, the proximal veins close, and the veins are refilled by blood passing through the perforators from the superficial system (Stemmer et al, 1980). During this cycle, in a normal leg, the distal valves of the deep veins and the valves of the perforators will ensure that the expelled blood can go in only one direction—upwards—back to the heart.

This 'pumping' action of the calf muscle causes the hydrostatic venous pressure in the ankle region to gradually fall until it reaches a steady state, usually about 30 mmHg in the deep veins and 40 mmHg in the superficial veins. If the subject then stands still, the pressure in both systems will slowly return to a stable value of about 90 mmHg, a process that usually takes about 20–30 seconds.

Blockage or damage to the venous system will cause disruption to normal blood flow, which may manifest itself in a number of different ways, according to the site and extent of the damage. If the valves in the perforators are damaged, some blood may be forced in the reverse direction, outwards into the superficial system, leading to the formation of varicosities. If the deep vessels are occluded by a thrombus, the pressure in the deep venous system may force blood out through the superficial system into the capillaries, causing venous flare and oedema from where fluid containing protein and red cells may leak into the surrounding tissue.

The application of external compression can help to minimise or reverse this process by forcing fluid from the interstitial spaces back into the vascular and lymphatic compartments. As the pressure within the veins of a standing subject is largely hydrostatic, it follows that the level of external pressure which is necessary to counteract this effect, will reduce progressively up the leg as the hydrostatic head is effectively reduced. For this reason, it is usual to ensure that external compression is applied in a graduated fashion, with the highest pressure at the ankle.

Much of the original information on the effects of compression on blood flow was obtained during the course of studies involving supine patients. Early work in this area was carried out by Stanton (1949), who used radiographic techniques to demonstrate that external compression of about 20 mmHg could increase the velocity of venous flow in the deep veins of the leg by about 45 per cent. Stanton postulated that this increase was due to a decrease in the cross-sectional area of the venous bed.

The importance of hydrostatic pressure was demonstrated by Sigel et al (1973), who showed that, relative to measurements taken with a patient in the horizontal position, lowering the feet by 10° decreased blood flow by an average of 53 per cent. In contrast, raising the feet by the same amount *increased* flow rate by 30 per cent.

Using a similar five-chambered pneumatic vinyl sleeve, Lawrence and Kakkar (1980) examined four different compression profiles and measured their effect upon deep venous velocity, calf muscle blood flow and subcutaneous tissue flow in supine patients in the 15° foot down tilt position. They found that graduated compression with 18 mmHg at the ankle produced a mean increase in deep venous velocity of about 75 per cent. Although higher levels of compression produced a further small increase in the mean velocity, 25 per cent of patients showed a reduction in deep venous velocity.[1]

Chant (1972) demonstrated that provided intravascular hydrostatic pressure is not exceeded, bandaging limits the formation of oedema, but does not increase vascular resistance to the detriment of blood flow.

The observed increase in blood velocity resulting from the application of rela-

---

[1] It is possible to calculate the theoretical hydrostatic pressure at various points along the leg of an individual in the 15° foot down tilt position. Depending upon the height of the subject, this will be in the order of 8 mmHg at the mid-thigh, 18 mmHg at the calf and 21 mmHg at the ankle. These values are in close agreement with those recommended by Sigel, and Lawrence and Kakkar.

tively low levels of external compression to supine individuals forms the basis of the current use of compression hosiery (anti-embolism stockings) for the prevention of deep vein thrombosis in certain groups of high risk patients who are confined to bed or undergoing surgery (Thomas 1992).

For ambulant patients who have greatly increased hydrostatic venous pressure in the lower leg, much higher levels of compression are required in order to produce a significant effect upon blood flow. This is reflected in the British Standard for compression hosiery (BS 6612:1985) which describes three different classes of stocking that provide levels of compression ranging from 14 to 35 mmHg at the ankle. The clinical indications for the use of these different profiles have been discussed previously by Scurr (1988), but it has been suggested by others that higher levels of compression, similar to those used in Germany, are likely to be of more value clinically (Burnand and Layer, 1986).

DEVELOPMENT OF EXTENSIBLE BANDAGES

Bandages in various forms have a history stretching back thousands of years to the time of the ancient Egyptians, who used simple woven fabrics often coated with adhesives, resins and other medicaments as dressings to aid wound healing. Unlike the majority of the bandages used today, these were made from non-extensible fabrics and would therefore have required considerable skill on the part of the users to ensure that they were applied correctly.

Early attempts at compression therapy for the treatment of leg ulcers were made in the seventeenth century, using rigid, lace-up stockings, as the bandages available at that time were not suitable for the application of sustained, controlled levels of pressure because of their inelastic nature. It was not until the middle of the nineteenth century that the first elasticated bandages containing natural rubber were manufactured and in 1878, Callender published a letter in the *Lancet*, describing the use of these materials in the management of varicose veins.

The first official British standards for bandages appeared in a supplement to the 1911 *British Pharmaceutical Codex* (*BPC*) which included a specification for crepe bandage, together with monographs for simple, non-extensible products such as calico, flannel, domette and open wove. As new products were developed over the years, additional monographs were introduced into the *BPC*, and when publication of the *BPC* ceased, many of these standards were transferred into the *British Pharmacopoeia*.

Despite differences in the structure and composition of the early bandages, the majority were produced from natural fibres such as cotton and wool by a weaving process, and in this respect they were essentially similar to the linen materials used by the ancient Egyptians thousands of years previously. Over the last 5–10 years, however, completely new products have been developed containing synthetic yarns made of polyamide and polyurethane, many of which are knitted rather than woven. These offer considerable advantages over the earlier bandages, being more comfortable (and thus easier to apply) with enhanced elastic properties. By careful selection of the elastomeric yarns used in their construction, the 'power' or strength of a bandage may be finely controlled, and thus for the first time it has become possible to design a bandage which will perform in a predetermined fashion in order to meet a specific clinical need.

IMPORTANT TERMS USED IN BANDAGING

In order to understand the science of bandaging, it is first necessary to become familiar with the following terms and definitions.

The **conformability** of a bandage determines its ability to follow the contours of a limb, and is governed by the density and extensibility of the fabric. The more open and extensible the structure, the more conformable the product is likely to be. As a general rule, knitted bandages tend to be more conformable than woven ones.

Extensibility determines the change in length that is produced when a bandage is subjected to an extending force. Extensibility is usually expressed in the form of a percentage which relates the stretched to the unstretched length. If the construction of the bandage is such that when it is stretched past a given point, the textile components prevent further extension, even though the elastomeric fibres may not have reached the limit of their elasticity, then **lock out** is said to have occurred.

Power or **modulus** describes the force that is required to bring about a specified increase in bandage length.

Elasticity determines the ability of a bandage subjected to an extending force (in the manner described above) to resist any change in length, and return to its original length once the applied force has been removed.

Support may be defined as the retention and control of tissue without the application of compression, and is usually provided to prevent the development of a deformity or a change in shape of a tissue mass due to swelling or sagging. Although non-extensible bandages can be used for this purpose, a product with a limited degree of extensibility is generally preferred as it is easier to apply.

Compression implies the deliberate application of pressure (see below) in order to produce a desired clinical effect. It is most commonly used to control oedema and reduce swelling in the treatment of venous disorders of the leg.

FACTORS INFLUENCING THE PRODUCTION OF SUB-BANDAGE PRESSURE

Sub-bandage pressure (which is generally measured in mmHg) may be calculated using the following formula, which has been derived from Laplace's equation.

$$P = \frac{TN \times 4630}{CW}$$

where P is the pressure (in mmHg), T is the bandage tension (in kgf), C is the circumference of the limb (in cm), W is the bandage width (in cm) and N is the number of layers applied. (*The Laplace equation more properly refers to the radius of curvature, but in the formula shown above this has been converted to limb circumference for practical purposes.*)

Because sub-bandage pressure is inversely proportional to limb circumference, it follows that a bandage applied with constant tension will exert different levels of pressure at various points on the leg. This will help to ensure the formation of a pressure gradient along the leg; for the average person the pressure at the calf will be lower than that produced at the ankle region because of the difference in circumference. Over the tibia, however, where the radius of curvature is relatively small, very high pressure may be generated. Further information on technical aspects of the performance of extensible bandages may be found elsewhere (Thomas, 1990).

In clinical practice, medical and nursing staff apply a compression bandage at the tension that they consider to be appropriate to the size and condition of the limb. This judgement is very subjective and, although a particular operator may produce reasonably consistent results from patient to patient, major differences will occur between the pressures achieved by different individuals, particularly if they are relatively inexperienced at bandage application (Logan et al, 1992). Operator technique is therefore a major factor in determining sub-bandage pressure and some attempts have been made to overcome this variation by printing geometrical designs upon bandages. These change shape when a predetermined level of tension is achieved. In this way, it is possible to exert some control over the tension with which a bandage is applied.

Because the pressure produced by successive layers of bandage are additive, it is possible to apply multiple layers of one or more products in order to achieve a desired clinical effect. This forms the basis of the so-called four-layer bandaging system described below.

CLASSIFICATION OF EXTENSIBLE BANDAGES

Although sub-bandage pressure is initially determined by the user, thereafter it is greatly influenced by the elastomeric properties of the fabric. In the past, a number of traditional bandages have been examined in clinical studies, which showed that the majority were unable to sustain clinically effective levels of pressure and therefore required frequent replacement (Raj et al, 1980; Tennant et al, 1988). Such studies are time-consuming, costly to perform, and are greatly influenced by operator technique and the method of pressure measurement.

A working party consisting of members of the surgical dressings industry, together with interested parties in the NHS, has recently devised a performance-based test method and classification system for extensible bandages, which may be used to characterise these materials in the laboratory and predict their ability to safely apply and maintain predetermined levels of compression on limbs of known dimensions. In particular, this test:

- Gives an indication of the degree of extension required to produce a predetermined level of compression.
- Determines the change in bandage tension (and hence sub-bandage pressure) that will occur as a result of small changes in limb circumference when the bandage is applied at the recommended extension.
- Provides assurance that when applied correctly, pressures greatly in excess of the target levels will not develop beneath the bandage in normal use.

This classification system, which now forms the basis of a draft British Standard, has also been adopted by the Drug Tariff.

In accordance with the classification system, bandages may be divided into the following groups:

Type 1: Lightweight Conforming Stretch Bandages

These have a simple dressing retention function, and usually contain lightweight elastomeric threads which impart a high degree of elasticity, but little power, to the bandage. There are many different types of these available, examples include Stayform™ (Robinsons), J Fast™ (Johnson & Johnson), Transelast™ (Lohmann) and Slinky™ (Cuxson Gerrard).

Type 2: Light Support Bandages

Products in this group, are also sometimes called short or minimal stretch bandages and include the familiar woven products of the *British Pharmacopoeia* such as crepe, cotton stretch and cotton crepe bandages together with numerous 'non-official' variations of these bandages, which are manufactured from cotton or cotton and viscose, and which show considerable variability in performance.

Compared with the compression bandages described below, light support or minimal stretch bandages have limited extensibility and elasticity, and tend to 'lock out' at relatively low levels of extension. It is this feature that enables them to be applied firmly over a joint to give support without generating significant levels of pressure.

Short stretch bandages are sometimes used in the treatment of venous leg ulcers on ambulant patients, particularly when a degree of ischaemia is suspected. In these situations the bandages form an inelastic covering to the leg, which tends to resist any change in the geometry of the calf muscle during exercise thereby increasing surface pressure and enhancing the action of the calf muscle pump. When the muscle relaxes this effect is partially reversed, producing a low level of residual compression. The pressure produced by short stretch bandages will also decrease significantly when the patient is at rest or the leg is elevated.

It follows therefore, that such products are *not* suitable for applying sustained compression to inactive individuals or for reducing existing oedema as they will not 'follow in' as a limb reduces in circumference.

Type 3: Compression Bandages

Compression implies the deliberate application of pressure and is most commonly employed to control oedema and reduce swelling in the treatment of venous disorders of the lower limb. These bandages have been divided into four groups according to their ability to produce predetermined levels of compression.

Type 3a: **Light compression bandages**, e.g. K crepe (Parema) and Tensolastic (Smith & Nephew) are able to provide *and maintain* low levels of pressure, up to 20 mmHg on an ankle of average dimensions. The clinical indications for products of this type include the management of superficial or early varices, and varicosis formed during pregnancy. In general, they are not suitable for controlling or reducing existing oedema, or for applying even low levels of pressure to very large limbs.

Type 3b: **Moderate compression bandages**, e.g. Veinopress™ (Steriseal), may be used to apply in the order of 30 mmHg on an ankle of average dimensions. They are indicated for the treatment of varicosis during pregnancy, varices of medium severity, the prevention and treatment of ulcers and the control of mild oedema.

Type 3c: **High compression bandages**, e.g. Tensopress™ (Smith & Nephew) and Setopress™ (Seton), may be used to apply high levels of compression in the order of 40 mmHg on an ankle of average dimensions. Indications for these bandages include the treatment of gross varices, post thrombotic venous insufficiency, and the management of leg ulcers and gross oedema in limbs of average circumference. Products in this category are not necessarily able to achieve these levels of pressure on very large limbs that have been further enlarged by the presence of oedema.

Type 3d: **Extra high performance compression bandages** are capable of applying pressures in excess of 50 mmHg. The power in the bandages is such that they can be expected to apply and sustain these pressures on even the largest and most oedematous limbs for extended periods of time. This group includes Elastic Web Bandage BP (Blue Line Webbing) and Tensopress™ (Smith & Nephew).

(All the pressures referred to above are based on the assumption that the bandage has been applied in the form of a spiral with a 50 per cent overlap between turns; effectively producing a double layer of bandage at any point on the limb.)

ADHESIVE/COHESIVE BANDAGES

In addition to the products described above, bandages are also available that are coated with adhesives or other substances that are designed to ensure they do not become displaced during use.

The most familiar products in this group are the Elastic Adhesive Bandages of the BP. These are made from woven cotton fabric coated with an adhesive mass which contains zinc oxide, rubber and natural resins, and these are used to provide support for fractured ribs, clavicles, injured joints and sports injuries.

Because zinc oxide/rubber based adhesives are known to cause skin reactions in some patients, products coated with synthetic adhesives have also been developed. Lestreflex™ (Seton) has an adhesive mass consisting of lead oleate and resin, and Poroplast™ (Scholl) is coated with an adhesive containing titanium dioxide. Other more lightweight adhesive bandages containing nylon or other synthetic yarns include Hapla-Band™ (Hinders-Leslies), Lite-Flex™ (Johnson & Johnson) and Veinoplast™ (Steriseal).

An extensible bandage coated with a hydrocolloid-based mass was shown in clinical studies to have an additional benefit upon hyperkeratotic skin and the eczema surrounding venous leg ulcers (Cherry et al, 1990). Called the Granuflex™ adhesive compression bandage it is now not actively promoted because of isolated reports of skin damage if the bandage is removed too frequently.

Cohesive bandages are designed to overcome some of the problems associated with the removal of adhesive products, for they have a special coating on their surface that enables the fabric to adhere to itself without sticking to the skin. This coating prevents overlapping turns from slipping under normal conditions of use. Cohesive bandages may be used in place of the adhesive products for many applications, but unlike the adhesive bandages they can be removed from the skin without causing pain or trauma.

The cohesive bandages currently on the market are Secure™ and Secure Forte™ (Johnson & Johnson), Cohepress™ (Steriseal), and Coban™ (3M).

TUBULAR BANDAGES

Tubular bandages are quick and easy to apply, and are often used as an alternative to roller bandages to provide pressure and support in the treatment of swollen legs. Unfortunately the levels of pressure that existing tubular bandages can produce are very limited and even a double layer will be unlikely to achieve more than 15 mmHg at the ankle. There is also a distinct possibility that the bandage may produce a slight reverse pressure gradient along the leg in some instances. Tubular bandages should therefore not be used as a substitute for a good compression bandage or as the sole means of applying pressure to an oedematous limb. Shaped tubular bandages may give a degree of graduated compression but the pressures produced by these bandages also fall short of the values that are required clinically.

CLINICAL ASPECTS OF COMPRESSION THERAPY

Although the importance of external compression in the treatment of venous leg ulcers has been recognised for many years, the majority of the bandages available historically have been unable to provide effective levels of sustained compression. This has been demonstrated both in the laboratory (Thomas et al, 1986) and in the clinical situation. Raj et al (1980) found that cotton bandages had to be reapplied every 6–8 hours if they were to achieve and maintain therapeutically active levels of pressure, and Tennant et al (1988) showed that over a four hour period, the pressure recorded beneath a crepe-type bandage fell by some 63 per cent. This compared with a 10 per cent drop beneath a competent compression bandage.

Barbenel et al (1990) compared the compression profiles produced by five different extensible bandages over a 1 hour period with particular reference to the bandage type and the application technique. They showed that according to the product applied, the calf pressure 30 minutes after application varied from 11 to 34 mmHg. In all cases, bandages applied in a figure of eight configuration resulted in pressures that were approximately 1.5–2 times those produced when the same bandages were applied in the form of a spiral with a 50 per cent overlap.

Using a specially designed pressure monitoring system, which consisted of a goniometer to detect the position of the lower leg (flexed or extended) and a sensor to measure sub-bandage pressure, Sockalingham et al (1990) were able to demonstrate differences between different types of bandages and also illustrate the effect of posture on sub-bandage pressure. During their investigations, both Barbenel et al (1990) and Sockalingham et al (1990) showed that the pressure produced by a short stretch bandage, Elastocrepe, was only one third of that produced by the Granuflex adhesive compression bandage.

The relative performance of three different bandaging systems was discussed by Callam et al (1991) who compared the effect of time and posture on the pressure profiles produced by an elastic bandage (Tensopress™) with a minimal stretch bandage (Elastocrepe™) and a non-elastic compression device consisting of concentric horizontal velcro bands (Circaid™). With a standing subject, all three regimens produced graduated compression for the duration of the study, but although the pressure beneath the elastic bandage remained relatively constant, the pressure beneath the non-elastic and minimal stretch regimen fell by about one third after 4 hours. In the lying position, the minimal stretch regimen also showed a loss or a reversal of graduation and the authors concluded that if this reduction in pressure were to continue, a question mark must be placed on the efficacy of the bandage system.

The importance of sustained compression in the treatment of chronic venous ulcers was demonstrated by Backhouse et al (1987) who described a trial in which they compared an occlusive dressing (Granuflex™) with a simple fabric dressing (NA™; Johnson & Johnson) in the treatment of 56 patients with chronic venous ulcers. A standard bandaging technique was used for both groups of patients, as follows. A layer of orthopaedic wadding (Velband™; Johnson & Johnson) was applied over the primary dressing, to act as an absorbent layer and distribute the pressure from the bandages that were applied subsequently. A layer of crepe bandage was then used to compress the Velband, and this was followed by a layer of Elset™ bandage (Seton) and a final layer of a cohesive bandage (Coban™; 3M). The pressure under these bandages was measured at four points between the medial malleolus and the knee in 16 volunteers. In each case, a gradual fall in pressure was recorded; from 42 mmHg at the ankle to 17 mmHg just below the knee.

As the healing rates in the two groups of patients was not significantly different, the authors stated that there was little benefit to be gained from the use of the occlusive dressing and concluded that "careful graduated compression bandaging achieves healing even in the majority of so-called 'resistant' chronic venous ulcers". However, it must be noted that only patients with small ulcers were included in this study (mean ulcer area was approximately 3 cm²).

Blair et al (1988) compared the pressure profiles produced by the four layer bandage system with those produced by an elastic adhesive bandage (Elastoplast™). In all cases, the pressures measured beneath the adhesive bandage were significantly lower than those recorded beneath the multi-component system. It was also reported that 74 per cent of ulcers that had failed to heal when dressed with a zinc paste bandage and an adhesive bandage healed within 12 weeks of the application of the four layer bandaging system. Practical advice on the application of the four-layer bandage has been published previously (Moffatt, 1992).

One specific group of patients who pose a particular problem in relation to the application of graduated compression are obese individuals with very large or awkward shaped legs. In order to achieve the required levels of compression on these patients, bandages must be applied with unusually high levels of tension, and many products are simply not suitable for this purpose. In these situations the selection of the appropriate bandages is essential if the treatment is to be successful (Thomas et al, 1992).

Compression bandaging is a powerful therapeutic tool, the importance and mechanisms of which are not widely understood. Like most powerful therapies, however, compression can also be misused with potentially very serious consequences for the patient. The effects of the application of excessive pressure following stripping of varices were described by Danner et al (1989) and Callam et al (1987) who recorded that the injudicious use of compression—in the form of bandages, hosiery or anti-embolism stockings—in limbs with occult arterial disease had apparently led to severe skin necrosis and, in a few instances, amputation. As a result, it was recommended that unless distal pulses of good volume could be detected, the ankle:brachial pressure index (ABPI) should be measured using Doppler ultrasound before compression therapy is commenced.

SUMMARY

- The application of external compression is a major factor in the successful treatment of venous leg ulcers, but the optimum levels of pressure required remain to be determined.
- If compression is applied by means of an extensible bandage, the pressure achieved will depend upon a number of factors, including the size and shape of the limb, the technique of the operator and the performance characteristics of the selected products.
- Many bandages are unable to sustain applied levels of compression and therefore rapidly become loose and displaced.
- Tubular bandages, although easier to apply, do not generally produce clinically effective levels of compression.
- The application of excessive pressure, or the use of compression bandages on ischaemic limbs, can impair blood flow which in extreme cases can lead to necrosis and amputation.
- Training in the selection and use of compression bandages should be provided to all clinical staff involved in the management of leg ulcers and other venous disorders.

Acknowledgements

Some of the content of this chapter has previously appeared in an article in the *Journal of Tissue Viability* and has been reproduced with their kind permission.

References

Backhouse C M, Blair S D, Savage A P, Walton J and McCollum C N (1987) Controlled trial of occlusive dressings in healing chronic venous ulcers. *British Journal of Surgery*, **74**: 626–627.

Barbenel J C, Sockalingham S and Queen D (1990) *In vivo* and laboratory evaluation of elastic bandages. *Care Science and Practice*, **8**: 72–74.

Blair S D, Wright D D I, Backhouse C M, Riddle E and McCollum C N (1988) Sustained compression and healing of chronic venous ulcers. *British Medical Journal*, **297**: 1159–1161.

Burnand K G and Layer G T (1986) Graduated elastic stockings. *British Medical Journal*, **293**: 224–225.

Callam M J, Ruckley C V, Dale J J and Harper D R (1987) Hazards of compression treatment of the leg: an estimate from Scottish surgeons. *British Medical Journal*, **295**: 1382.

Callam M J, Haiart D, Farouk M, Brown D, Prescott R J and Ruckley C V (1991) Effect of time and posture on pressure profiles obtained by three different types of compression. *Phlebology*, **6**: 79–84.

Chant A D B (1972) The effect of posture, exercise and bandage pressure on the clearance of ^{24}Na from the subcutaneous tissues of the foot. *British Journal of Surgery*, **59**: 552–555.

Cherry G W, Cameron J, Cherry C and Ryan T J (1990) Clinical comparison of a new adhesive compression bandage with other treatments. *Care Science and Practice*, **8**: 80–82.

Danner R, Partanen K, Partanen J and Kettunen K (1989) Iatrogenic compartment syndrome, a follow-up of four cases caused by elastic bandages. *Clinical Neurology & Neurosurgery,* **91**: 37–43.

Lawrence D and Kakkar V V (1980) Graduated, static external compression of the lower limb: a physiological assessment. *British Journal of Surgery,* **67**: 119–121.

Logan R A, Thomas S, Harding E F and Collyer G J (1992) A comparison of sub-bandage pressures produced by experienced and inexperienced bandagers. *Journal of Wound Care,* **1**(3): 23–26.

Moffatt C J (1992) Compression bandaging—the state of the art. *Journal of Wound Care,* 1(1): 45–50.

Raj T B, Goddard M and Makin G S (1980) How long do compression bandages maintain their pressure during ambulatory treatment of varicose veins. *British Journal of Surgery,* **67**: 122–124.

Scurr J (1988) Why use elastic hosiery? *Pharmaceutical Journal,* **240**: 410–411.

Sigel B, Edelstein A L, Felix W R and Memhardt C R (1973) Compression of the deep venous system of the lower leg during inactive recumbancy. *Archives of Surgery,* **106**: 38–43.

Sockalingham S, Barbenel J C and Queen D (1990) Ambulatory monitoring of the pressures beneath compression bandages. *Care Science and Practice,* **8**: 75–79.

Stanton J R (1949) Acceleration of linear flow in deep veins of lower extremity of man by local compression. *Journal of Clinical Investigation,* **28**: 553–558.

Stemmer R, Marescaux J and Furderer C (1980) Compression treatment of the lower extremities particularly with compression stockings. *Dermatologist,* **31**: 355–365.

Tennant W G, Park K G M and Ruckley C V (1988) Testing compression bandages. *Phlebology,* **3**: 55–61.

Thomas S, Wilde L G and Loveless P (1986) Performance profiles of extensible bandages. In: *Phlebology '85,* eds Negus D and Jantet G, pp. 667–670. London: Libbey.

Thomas S (1990) Bandages and bandaging. In: *Wound Management and Dressings.* London: The Pharmaceutical Press.

Thomas S (1992) *Graduated External Compression and the Prevention of Deep Vein Thrombosis.* Bridgend: Surgical Materials Testing Laboratory.

Thomas S, Fear M and Logan R A (1992) Compression therapy in an obese patient. *Journal of Wound Care,* **1**(1): 19–20.

7

The Art and Science of

Bandaging

INTRODUCTION

Bandaging is used to retain dressings, restrict joint motion and as a treatment in its own right for venous ulceration. The teaching of the art of flat bandaging has suffered from the advent of the tubular bandage, which can be used to hold a dressing in the most awkward position. Tubular bandages can also be employed in the treatment of venous ulceration, but the majority of practitioners prefer to rely on the application of a compression bandage. Support stockings are used in some centres to provide the compression necessary to heal venous leg ulcers. However, this is not widely accepted due to the need for accurate stocking fitting, the difficulty of applying stockings over dressings, and the tendency of the stocking to become soiled with exudate.

Successful bandaging depends on the choice of an appropriate bandage and its effective application. Research indicates that few nurses understand the principles behind bandaging (Magazinovic et al, 1993) and it is no surprise that this results in poor choice of bandages and their ineffective application (Magazinovic et al, 1993; Millard et al, 1986).

Bandage choice and application are governed by scientific principles. In the previous chapter, Thomas has described different types of bandage, their evaluation and indications for clinical practice. This chapter will describe the principles behind bandage application, methods of bandage application in common use and various techniques for adapting bandage application to particular situations.

THE AIM OF BANDAGE APPLICATION

The aim of applying a compression bandage to a leg with a venous ulcer is to heal the ulcer. The exact pressure required is still a matter of debate. Clearly the required pressure must vary according to circumstances. However, research indicates that for a typical venous ulcer there should be 30–40 mmHg compression at the ankle, reducing at the calf to around 15–20 mmHg (Stemmer, 1969). These pressures have been shown to heal ulcers but an optimal pressure profile has not been determined. As the majority of nurses have no access to pressure measurement devices it is important that bandaging technique is assessed clinically, gathering clues from the patient and their leg. To this end, the nurse should:

- Ask the patient to report any discomfort.
- Check that the bandage has stayed in place.
- Observe the leg for the formation of oedema where the bandage has been loose, or for redness and ridging where the bandage has been too tight.

Thomas has described how sub-bandage pressure is influenced by the type of bandage and the way in which it is applied (Laplace's law—see chapter 6). In general, the greater the extension of the bandage, the more layers applied and the smaller the radius of curvature of the leg, the higher the pressure generated. An analogy is the discomfort felt when carrying a heavy bag; your fingers are less comfortable if the bag is very heavy, if there are many bags or if you try to carry the bag on one finger instead of the whole hand. Thus the pressure applied to the leg can be varied by choice of bandage, and/or by modifying the tension and the numbers of layers employed. However, the pressure under a bandage, and therefore its therapeutic effect, does not remain constant. Immediately after application the pressure exerted by the bandage falls (Raj et al, 1980) and the pressure is also affected by the posture of the patient (Sockalingham et al, 1990). The decrease of pressure with time is dependent on bandage characteristics and the method of application (Thomas et al, 1980). Therefore the actual pressure under a bandage is of major clinical importance. It has been measured by investigators interested in evaluating bandage performance in the clinical environment and in correlating that performance with therapeutic benefit.

SUB-BANDAGE PRESSURE MEASUREMENT

Various ways of measuring the pressure exerted by a bandage both in the laboratory and on patients have been described (Robertson et al, 1980; Dawson and Kidd, 1988; Sockalingham et al, 1990). None is ideal and the results obtained with one method are not directly comparable with those obtained with another. In the UK, stocking pressures are regulated by a British Standard (BS6612;1985) and their pressures are measured in the laboratory using tensometers and leg formers (the Hatra method), again with little comparability with results achieved by other bench tests, e.g. Instron or Hohenstein (Dawson and Kidd, 1988).

Pressures may be estimated, rather than actually measured, using Laplace's relationship between pressure, tension, layers and leg radius. When bandaging a leg one does not know the tension, or force, in the bandage but can assume that tension increases with increasing extension. Thus one can calculate the relative pressures at the ankle and the calf and this shows whether a gradient has been achieved (see figure 7.1).

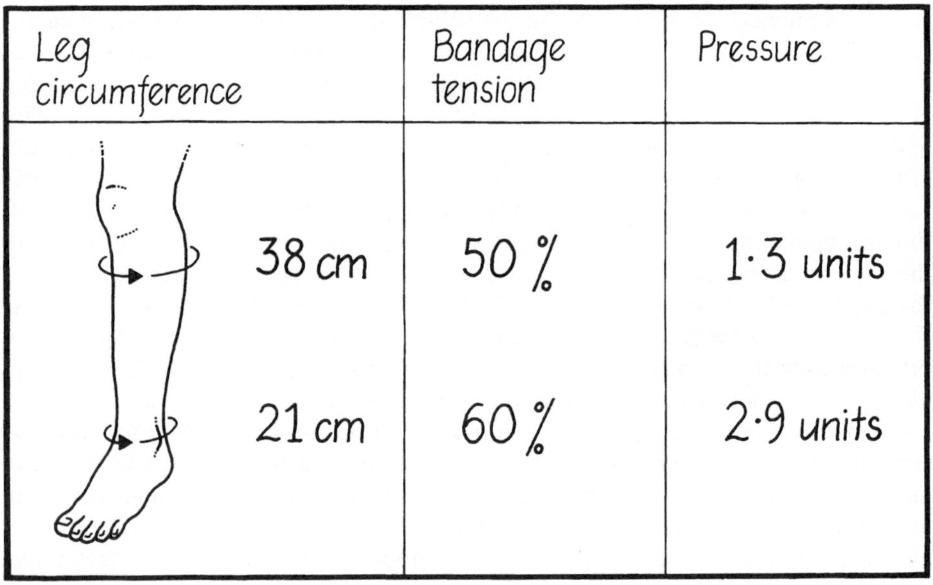

Leg circumference	Bandage tension	Pressure
38 cm	50 %	1·3 units
21 cm	60 %	2·9 units

Fig 7.1 Calculating pressure gradient

ESTIMATION OF PRESSURE GRADIENT USING THE LAW OF LAPLACE

- Mark a bandage at 10 cm intervals using a marker pen.
- Measure the circumference of a volunteer's leg at the narrowest part of the ankle and at the widest part of the calf.
- Apply the bandage in a spiral with 50 per cent overlap, and measure the distance between two lines at the ankle and between two lines at the calf.
- Calculate the bandage extension at the ankle and the calf thus;

Extension (%) = 10 × {(new distance between pen marks − 10 cm)}

- Use extension and circumference to estimate the pressure gradient along leg as follows:

CALF:	Circumference	=	38 cm
	Bandage extension	=	50% (i.e. 10 × {15−10})
Calculation:	$P = 50/38$	=	1.3 times a constant (k)

ANKLE:	Circumference	=	21 cm
	Bandage extension	=	60% (i.e. 10 × {16−10})
Calculation:	$P = 60/21$	=	2.9 times a constant (k)

The value of the constant depends on the bandage used and the numbers of bandage layers applied. If there is an even number of layers applied then in this example the bandage pressure is graduated from ankle to calf.

The commonest method of measuring sub-bandage pressure is by placing an air or fluid-filled balloon on the leg prior to bandaging. The balloon is connected to a pressure transducer or in the simplest devices, a mercury manometer (Robertson et al, 1980).

After bandaging, the pressure at the balloon site is read from the manometer. Unfortunately, the interpretation of the reading is not necessarily straightforward. Laplace's law states that the sub-bandage pressure is dependent on the radius of the site being considered. If the balloon itself distorts the site of measurement then the pressure reading will not accurately reflect the pressure exerted without the balloon. The size of the balloon will also influence the resolution of the results. If the balloon is large, then the pressure reading is effectively an average of the pressure over the area of the balloon and pressure gradients will be masked. An ideal pressure sensor is therefore small in diameter and thickness.

Commercial pressure monitors based on this principle include the Oxford Pressure monitor, the Borgnis Medical Stocking tester and the Strathclyde pressure monitor. These are all relatively expensive and the nurse may only encounter them at bandaging workshops or at training courses. Thus it is important to be able to evaluate one's own bandaging technique without these devices. The technique described above may be used. It is also important when removing a bandage, to assess the effect that it has had on the patient's leg. The leg may be imprinted with tell-tale signs such as indentations, chafing and signs of pressure damage; the ulcer may demonstrate poor healing, there may be sensitivity reactions to components of the bandage, and there may be oedema, all of which indicate problems with bandaging technique (see plate 11). Alternatively, absence of these signs together with good healing progress suggest satisfactory bandaging.

CHOICE OF BANDAGE

There are various, measurable ways of describing bandages, e.g. by their degree of elasticity, whether they are long-stop or short-stop, adhesive or cohesive. Other characteristics such as bandage compliance and patient comfort are less easy to measure but are of practical importance. The preceding chapter has described bandage classification and in this chapter the clinical relevance of these bandage types and application techniques will be outlined.

Sub-bandage pressure is influenced by bandage type and construction (Thomas et al, 1980), by the posture of the patient (Sockalingham et al, 1990), the time since application (Raj et al, 1980), washing the bandage (Dale et al, 1983), the method of application, the number of layers, muscular activity and the curvature of the limb (Thomas, 1990).

EFFECT OF WASHING

Washing a crepe bandage will reduce its elasticity as the crimped fibres which give the bandage its elasticity will not regain their crimped state (Dale et al, 1983). Bandages containing artificial elastic fibres, e.g. Lycra or Elastane, wash well and can be washed up to 20 times without loss of elasticity. This means they are more economical in the long term despite the initial cost. Cotton crepe BP bandages (e.g. Elastocrepe™; Smith & Nephew) exerted 76 per cent of their original sub-bandage pressure after only one wash in one study (Dale et al, 1983). It is important to note that the artificial fibres must be washed according to the manufacturer's instructions. Boil washing will damage the elastic fibres.

DECREASE IN PRESSURE WITH TIME

All bandages lose their pressure over time, necessitating frequent reapplication to sustain therapeutic pressures (Raj et al, 1980). Cohesive (which stick to themselves only) and adhesive (stick to themselves and to the skin) bandages may maintain their pressures better than other bandages, but have the disadvantage of not always being washable (Sockalingham et al, 1990).

PRESSURE VARIATION WITH POSTURE

Long-stretch (or elastic) bandages are able to 'give' when the tissue below them changes shape, and to return to their original extension. Thus when a patient moves from a sitting to a standing posture, there is only a small rise in pressure. Short-stretch (or inelastic) bandages form a firm 'skin' over the leg, however, and when the calf muscle contracts the bandage cannot yield and therefore the pressure under the bandage will increase significantly (see figure 7.3). These pressure changes, which occur as the patient becomes increasingly upright and during walking, may be therapeutic by enhancing the action of the calf pump. The fact that the inelastic bandages exert high pressures only during walking or in the upright posture may make them safer for patients whose ulcers are complicated by arterial impairment, although of course when there is marked arterial impairment elastic compression should not be applied. Inelastic bandages are used widely in the German-speaking countries while elastic bandages are preferred in the UK and France. A recent study has shown the healing rates achieved with elastic bandages was significantly higher than those with inelastic bandages (Callam et al, 1992).

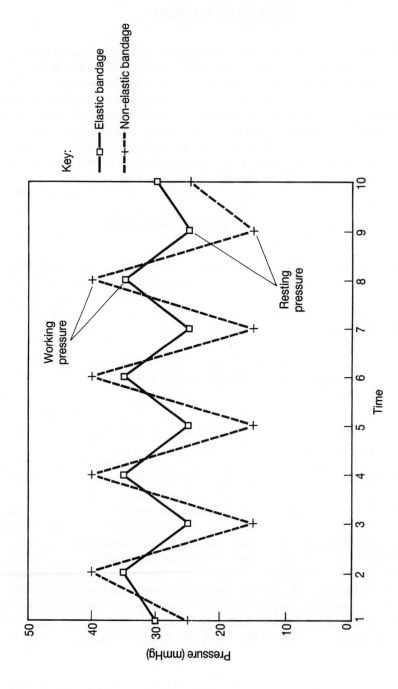

Fig 7.2 Pressure variation with movement; elastic and non-elastic bandages

BANDAGING TECHNIQUES

The leg is covered from the base of the metatarsals to the tibial plateau in each recommended bandaging technique. If the bandage is begun more proximally, the tissues beyond the bandage will become oedematous. The grossly oedematous leg is particularly vulnerable to bandage damage and it is recommended that oedema is reduced by a period of bed rest with high elevation of the limb prior to application of a compression bandage (Dale and Gibson, 1993).

In order to allow the maximum range of motion of the ankle joint, the leg should be bandaged with the ankle in a neutral position. Bandaging for a venous ulcer is usually done with the patient seated and the leg dependent. Post-sclerotherapy, bandaging is done with the patient supine and the leg raised. This drains the leg and results in higher pressures once the patient is seated or standing due to the increase in the volume of the leg. Likewise the volume of the leg increases during the day and therefore a bandage may increase in tightness towards the evening (Blair et al, 1988).

Simple Spiral

Advantages of this method
1. Simple to apply.
2. Method recommended for strong compression bandages which may cause skin damage if applied in a figure of eight.
3. Patients may be trained to reapply their own bandages.

Disadvantages of this method
1. Does not provide as much compression as the figure of eight method.
2. Bandage position is less well held, the bandages tending to slip down the leg if non-adhesive or the leg is 'champagne bottle' shaped.

Simple spiral is the simplest technique and the majority of elastic bandages are applied in this way. Other methods are based on this and so it will be described in detail. As with all techniques the bandage is applied with the roll outwards (see figure 7.4). A 50 per cent overlap results in the leg being covered with two layers of bandage from ankle to knee. By increasing the amount of overlap to 66 or 75 per cent, three or four layers can be applied. It is important to keep the degree of overlap constant along the leg. The layers of bandage are kept to a minimum on the foot, so that patients can wear their normal footwear and thus walk normally, utilising the calf pump.

The Foot

This part of the bandaging remains the same whether a spiral or figure of eight technique is being used. The full bandage extension, to be used for the rest of the leg, is not applied to the foot which is well-supported by footwear and is a bony structure which will not tolerate high pressures over the thin skin. The manufacturer's instruction leaflets, supplied with the bandage, should be consulted for additional information.

1. The first turn encircles the ball of the foot and anchors the bandage in place (plate 12).
2. The next turn takes the bandage to the point of the heel and back to the front of the foot ready to cover the arch of the foot in turn 3 (plate 13).
3. The third turn encircles the rest of the foot and returns to the Achilles tendon from where the straight part of the leg can be approached (plate 14).

The Rest of the Leg (plates 15 and 16)

4. At this point the bandage can be extended to its required extension. The bandage is then applied by unrolling the bandage to a length suitable for wrapping around the leg, extending it to the required extension, and then placing it on the leg so that 50 per cent of the previous turn is covered. When using cohesive or adhesive bandages it is important to release the bandage from the roll and then relax the bandage fully before extending it to the required extension. Otherwise one may apply these bandages at full stretch, straight from the roll, resulting in extremely high pressures. The bandage is passed from one hand to the other to achieve an even extension and overlap up the leg as far as the tibial plateau, where the bandage is finished so that the knee joint is not impeded. In obese patients, the knee joint may be difficult to locate and it may help to ask the patient to bend the knee in order to determine its position.

Any excess bandage should be cut off rather than wound around the leg since extra layers will cause a tourniquet effect. Pins or metal fasteners should not be used due to the possibility that they may damage the skin of either the bandaged or the other leg. Adhesive tape should be used to secure the bandage effectively.

Figure of Eight, Spica or Criss-cross Method

Advantages
1. The degree of compression achieved with an equivalent bandage is higher than the simple spiral.
2. Champagne bottle shaped legs are easier to bandage this way.
3. The bandage is more likely to remain in position.

Disadvantages
1. More difficult to apply than the simple spiral.
2. There may be a concentration of pressure where the bandage layers cross over and this may lead to pressure necrosis over tendon, or bone such as the tibial crest.

The foot is covered in the same way as described for the spiral technique (plates 12–14). The first turn of the bandage above the ankle is applied up the lateral aspect of the leg, straight along the back of the leg and then downwards along the medial aspect. The next turn along the back of the leg is offset by 1/2 bandage width and the following turns are placed accordingly. The pattern repeats up the leg to the tibial plateau (see plate 17).

MODIFICATIONS FOR PARTICULAR BANDAGES

Paste

These bandages are always used in conjunction with a compression bandage so their use is primarily as a dressing; however, they also improve the maintenance of compression of some bandages and can augment the pressures achieved; in effect converting any overlying bandage to a non-stretch system (Dale et al, 1983). The main disadvantage of paste bandages is the high rate of allergy engendered. For this reason, the first application of a paste bandage should always be followed up by a visit or phone call from the nurse to check that there is no sensitivity reaction.

Paste bandages are completely inelastic and are applied in such a manner that the leg does not become constricted when the leg swells and the bandage dries out. Although there is no evidence of the need to apply them discontinuously, they are traditionally applied with frequent folds in the fabric or by cutting them into strips. Dale and Gibson (1993) recommend the former as the folds can be placed along the tibial crest as a protection from pressure damage. As this method requires manual dexterity, the infrequent user may prefer to cut the bandage after every circumference of the leg.

The Short-stretch Bandage

These bandages can be stretched by up to 90 per cent of their original length. This type of bandage is not widely used in the UK although some workers have reported its effectiveness (Charles, 1991). The manufacturer's information leaflets should be consulted for the recommended method of application.

ASPECTS OF TECHNIQUE: EXTENSION AND OVERLAP

Bandage Extension

Manufacturer's information leaflets should be consulted for the recommended extension. It is worth while practising achieving the required extensions with each bandage until one is familiar with it. This can be done by marking the new bandage with felt pen at 10 cm intervals.

Once one has stretched the bandage, the extension achieved is calculated thus:

% Extension = (Distance between pen marks − 10 cm) × 10

For example, a bandage stretched to 12 cm has [(12 − 10) × 10] = **20 per cent extension**.

For some bandages a medium extension is recommended for legs of average size and a greater extension for very large legs, e.g. Tensopress™ (Smith & Nephew).

As the ability to gauge extension is not easily acquired, symbols have been printed on some bandages in order to indicate when the desired extension has been attained. For example, Setopress™ (Seton) and Biflex™ (Thuasne, France) feature a rectangle which becomes a square at the desired extension. Other symbols include an oval (which becomes a circle at the critical extension) which can be stamped onto a bandage. According to Laplace's law, if the extension of the bandage is kept constant, the changing shape of the patient's leg will result in a pressure gradient from ankle to knee. This is the principle behind the marking of bandages with tension indicators.

Common Problems

When handing the bandage over from the right to the left hand or vice versa, it is important to maintain a constant tension. A common mistake is for the bandager to increase extension up the leg (due to the increase in leg circumference) or to over-extend the bandage at the top of the leg due to a fear of running out of bandage (Dale et al, 1983). Either will cause a tourniquet effect. Raj et al (1980) commented that there was also a tendency for a tourniquet to form at the point where two bandages were joined.

Overlap

Bandage extension alone will not control the pressure under a chosen bandage. The number of layers and therefore the overlap is of great importance. Two layers will exert approximately twice the pressure of a single layer and therefore damage can be caused with apparently innocuous bandages. The bandager may choose to vary the number of layers during the treatment and one author describes this as a method for gradually increasing the amount of compression tolerated by the patient (Hansson and Swanbeck, 1988). Most practitioners, however, are content to apply bandages in one of the standard fashions.

An overlap of 50 per cent is generally used and many bandages have lines along their length to indicate to the bandager when 50 per cent of the preceding layer has been covered. In the absence of these lines the bandager can check on the overlap obtained by measuring the depth of bandage still exposed after application (see plate 18).

PROBLEM LEGS

The 'champagne bottle' shaped leg is common in patients with long standing chronic venous insufficiency. The gaiter area is hard, indurated and contracted where there has been scarring and deposition of fibrin. Above it the calf muscle bulk causes an abrupt increase in the circumference of the leg which is particularly difficult to bandage.

Tips for Dealing with Champagne-bottle Legs

1. Pad the narrow part of the leg with plenty of gamgee or orthopaedic wadding to make the leg more cone shaped (see plate 19).
2. Use a figure of eight or criss cross technique as they are less prone to slippage.
3. Consider using a 7.5 cm bandage in preference to the standard 10 cm bandage as this may be easier to fit to the steep part of the leg.
4. Use an adhesive bandage or fix the bandage layers with a cohesive bandage to prevent slippage.

The Very Large Leg

Laplace's Law states that there is a reduction in pressure as leg circumference increases, therefore large legs may not receive sufficient compression unless the basic techniques are amended.

1. Consider using a Type 3d bandage instead of a Type 3c bandage (see Thomas's classification of bandages, chapter 6).
2. Use a figure of eight (spica or criss cross) technique.
3. Read the bandage instructions carefully to see if manufacturers recommend a higher extension for larger legs.
4. Consider using additional layers of bandages to achieve the pressure required, e.g. a Type 3c bandage plus a shaped tubigrip or a layered system as described by the Charing Cross team (Blair et al, 1988).

'I Can't Wear Tight Bandages'

If the patient is intolerant of all compression then one may need to reconsider the diagnosis or check for infection. If the ulcer is purely venous you can help the patient participate in treatment by using compression hosiery. An improvement in ulcer condition generally increases patient compliance.

A compression bandage with a final layer of a shaped tubular bandage (SSB™, Seton or Flexishape™, Smith & Nephew) may permit the patient to feel in control of the compression on his/her leg. They can be shown how to remove the top layer in the evening if the bandage is slightly uncomfortable and to reapply it first thing in the morning. This approach may be useful in the patient who is reluctant to tolerate high compression throughout 24 hours.

The Thin Leg

This leg experiences a higher pressure for a given bandage tension than a larger leg (due to Laplace's Law) and is prone to pressure damage. There may be little or no change in circumference between the ankle and the calf thus the nurse cannot rely on Laplace's Law to graduate the pressure along the leg.

1. Protect the leg with a paste bandage or with a soft padding.
2. Decrease the bandage extension as you approach the top of the leg in order to graduate the pressure.
3. Be especially vigilant for signs of pressure necrosis.

MINIMISING PRESSURE NECROSIS

The fact that pressure damage is an under-reported problem was illustrated by Callam's survey among Scottish surgeons (Callam et al, 1987). Pressure-induced damage may lead to amputation in extreme cases and therefore one should always consider the possibility of pressure damage when applying a compression bandage. The first safeguard is an accurate diagnosis. Applying a compression bandage to an ischaemic leg is obviously dangerous as arterial inflow will be impeded. Refer to chapter 4 for an account of the nursing assessment of the patient with leg ulceration. Once it is clear that an ulcer is not complicated by arterial, diabetic, rheumatoid or neurological disease, then one should consider the shape of the leg. Laplace's law states that the pressure at a point is inversely proportional to the radius of curvature of the surface. Thus thin legs and any part of the leg with a small curve will have high pressures exerted on them. Thin legs may be protected by applying a layer of orthopaedic wadding under the compression bandage. As this is not yet available to all nurses then one may have to choose a bandage for the leg which will minimise the chance of damage. A strong compression bandage will generally be accompanied by manufacturer's instructions recommending the size of legs which can be treated safely – usually of the order of 18 cm circumference. For legs with ankles of circumference less than 18 cm, a medium-strength bandage must be used instead, e.g. class 2, cotton crepe (e.g. Elastocrepe™, Smith & Nephew) instead of a class 3c bandage (e.g. Setopress, Seton). One may also consider using an inelastic bandage which will only exert high pressures when the patient is upright. The lower resting pressures allow a safety margin.

Vulnerable Areas

The tendons, tibial crest and the malleoli are all bony prominences with small radii of curvature and hence are at risk of pressure necrosis. Regular, frequent inspection of these areas at dressing changes should prevent significant deterioration of the skin condition. Any skin breaks on these areas should be regarded as indicative of pressure damage particularly if there is no new ulcer development elsewhere on the leg. Strategies to protect these areas are based on the concept of smoothing out the pressure at these points by flattening the curvature of the leg. This can be done with foam pads, either fashioned out of chiropody foam, or supplied already shaped, or with orthopaedic wadding. Foam 'polos' are particularly useful to protect the malleoli or rheumatoid nodules on the feet (see plate 20) and can be reused if not soiled.

Around Dressings

Pressure damage may also occur at the edge of a thick dressing (see plate 21). For this reason gauze swabs or other absorptive material should be placed so as to avoid thick edges. If modern dressings are being used one may choose one with a bevelled edge or trim the dressing so that the edges do not fall on vulnerable parts of the leg.

SUMMARY

This chapter has presented information to help the nurse select and apply a compression bandage effectively. There is evidence that nurses do not extract the full potential from the bandages now available, and it is hoped that greater education will allow the nurse to develop the skill of compression bandaging.

Pressure measurement is important for the evaluation of bandages and for nurse training, but as the various methods used do not produce equivalent results, their limitations have been described. As pressure monitors are not widely used in training, the majority of nurses need to be able to assess their own skills objectively and some guidelines have been given.

Both the simple spiral and figure of eight bandaging techniques are described along with hints for bandaging problem legs.

Pressure necrosis is best avoided by accurate diagnosis and the avoidance of compression in legs with substantial arterial disease. Vigilance during dressing changes is important in the detection of pressure-induced damage. Vulnerable patients such as those with thin legs and sharp bony prominences can be protected from pressure damage by the judicious use of padding materials.

References

Blair S D, Wright D D I, Backhouse C M, Riddle E and McCollum C N (1988) Sustained compression and healing of chronic venous ulcers. *British Medical Journal*, **297**: 1159–1161.

Callam M J, Ruckley C V, Dale J J and Harper D R (1987) Hazards of compression treatment of the leg: an estimate from Scottish surgeons. *British Medical Journal*, **295**: 1382.

Callam M J, Harper D R, Brown D, Gibson B, Prescott R J and Ruckley C V (1992) Lothian and Forth Valley Leg Ulcer Healing Trial. Part 1: Elastic versus non-elastic bandaging in the treatment of chronic leg ulceration. *Phlebology*, **7**: 136–141.

Charles H (1991) Compression healing of ulcers. *Journal of District Nursing*, **September**: 4–8.

Dale J J, Callam M J and Ruckley C V (1983) How efficient is a compression bandage? *Nursing Times*, **November**, 49–51.

Dale J J and Gibson B (1993) Systematic care brings results. *Professional Nurse*, **Suppl 8**(5).

Dawson G A and Kidd B (1988) An analysis of two indirect methods of measuring compression. *Swiss Medicine*, **10**(4a): 85–86.

Hansson C and Swanbeck G (1988) Regulating the pressure under compression bandages for venous leg ulcers. *Acta Dermatogia Venereologia (Stockholm)*, **68**: 245–249.

Magazinovic N, Phillips-Turner J and Wilson G V (1993) Assessing nurses' knowledge of bandages and bandaging. *Journal of Wound Care*, **2**(2): 97–101.

Millard L G, Bleacher A and Fentem P H (1986) The pressure at which nursing staff apply compression bandages when treating patients with varicose ulcers. In: *Phlebology '85*, eds Negus D and Jantet G, pp. 682–685. London: Libbey.

Raj T B, Goddard M and Makin G S (1980) How long do compression bandages maintain their pressure during ambulatory treatment of varicose veins? *British Journal of Surgery*, **67**: 122–124.

Robertson J C, Shah J, Amos H, Druett J E and Gisby J (1980) An interface pressure sensor for routine clinical use. *Engineering in Medicine*, **9**: 151–156.

Sockalingham S, Barbenel J C and Queen D (1990) Ambulatory monitoring of the pressures beneath compression bandages. *Care Science and Practice*, **8**(2): 75–79.

Stemmer R (1969) Ambulatory elastocompressive treatment of the lower extremities with elastic stockings. *Zeitschift fur Aerztlichl Fortbildung*, **3**: 1–8.

Thomas, S, Dawes C and Hay P (1980) A critical evaluation of some extensible bandages in current use. *Nursing Times*, **76**: 1123–1126.

Thomas S (1990) Bandages and bandaging: the science behind the art. *Care Science and Practice*, **8**: 56–60.

8

Prevention of Re-ulceration

There is an urgent need for the prevention of ulceration, because as Browse (1983) states:

"Once an ulcer appears, the skin has been irretrievably damaged and the chance of restoring the skin to normal has been lost. With post-phlebitic ulcers the case is not one of 'prevention is better than cure', we must prevent because we have no cure".

RECURRENCE RATES

Leg ulcer recurrence rates are high and ulcers can recur over long periods of time, particularly if the cause is left untreated. Callam et al (1985) described the natural history of venous ulcers using data from a survey of 600 patients with 827 ulcerated legs, 76 per cent of which had a venous component. Of the 827 ulcerated legs, 555 (67 per cent) already had recurrent ulcers; 287 (35 per cent) had experienced four or more episodes of ulceration, 268 (32 per cent), two or three episodes, and in just 272 (33 per cent) cases the patient was suffering from a leg ulcer for the first time.

In 1981, a leg ulcer survey conducted by Cornwall et al (1986) in the Harrow Health District identified 357 patients with 424 ulcerated limbs. During 1988, a follow-up study was undertaken by Cornwall et (1989) al to investigate the long-term outcome. Of the original 357 patients, 35 per cent were known to be alive, 54 per cent had died, 9 per cent had moved out of the area and 2 per cent could not be traced. Of those patients known to be alive, 112 agreed to provide information to the follow-up study. The original ulcers had healed in 92 per cent of these patients. However, there had been at least one recurrence of ulceration on the same limb, in 53 per cent of patients where the original ulcer had healed. A further 6 per cent of patients had a recurrence on the other limb. In those patients with a recurrence on the same limb, 60 per cent had a single recurrence, 25 per cent had experienced two to three recurrences and 15 per cent had four or more recurrences (the maximum number was eight). What was particularly striking was that use of compression hosiery appeared to have conferred no particular benefit. This may have been because the compression hosiery available on the FP10 before April

1988 was inadequate. Monk and Sarkany (1982) reviewed the outcome of 39 patients admitted to hospital for the treatment of venous ulcers. They found that half of the ulcers recurred within 3 months of discharge and two thirds within 1 year.

TRIALS TO PREVENT RECURRENCE

It is believed that compression hosiery helps to prevent the recurrence of venous ulcers; however, the contribution of compression hosiery has not been adequately evaluated. Ethically it would be extremely difficult to conduct a randomised controlled trial comparing compression therapy with no compression, as weaker evidence from other types of study, and expert opinion deems compression to be an essential component of ulcer prevention. Several centres have documented the results of the follow-up of patients wearing compression stockings for healed venous ulcers. Recurrence rates of 16–30 per cent are typical, despite regular monitoring of patients and accurate fitting of the compression hosiery. Cherry (1986) found that 30 per cent of 136 patients with healed ulcers recurred despite regular follow-up. Where there had been breakdown of lesions, lack of compliance or the patient's inability to put on the stockings were regarded as major factors responsible for recurrence. Mayberry et al (1991) followed up 73 patients for 30 months. Fifty eight patients (79 per cent) continued to be compliant with stockings and 15 patients were non-compliant. Total ulcer recurrence in patients who were compliant was 16 per cent. All patients who were non-compliant had recurrent ulceration within 36 months. Dinn and Henry (1992) reported a 5 year follow-up of 126 patients who had undergone successful healing of venous ulcers by injection sclerotherapy and compression hosiery. Of the 126 patients, 21 dropped out, 72 patients remained healed and 33 (26 per cent) patients experienced ulcer recurrence; injury being a causative factor in nine cases.

In 1991, Nash evaluated the factors influencing recurrence after standard surgical procedures and the use of fitted compression stockings. He followed up 90 patients for a period of 3 years. Forty two patients had superficial vein incompetence whilst 48 had deep vein involvement. Only one patient in the superficial vein group developed a recurrence whilst 15 patients in the deep vein group either failed to heal or recurred within 18 months. Deep vein involvement was also identified as a factor delaying healing by Skene et al (1992). They devised a prognostic index to predict time to healing. Four factors influenced healing rates; age, ulcer duration, ulcer size and deep vein involvement. Using this information, patients can be stratified into low, medium and high risk groups. Those patients with deep vein involvement are far more likely to have ulcers that are slow to heal or fail to heal and therefore pose a high risk of recurrence.

COMPRESSION HOSIERY

History

The use of compression on the legs as a treatment for venous disorders can be traced back to the ancient Egyptians. Richard Wiseman (1676) introduced a rigid lace-up stocking as a method of compressing a leg affected by leg ulcers. The first elastic stocking was developed in Nottingham in the early 1840s by Taberer (Davison, 1970).

Function

Compression therapy has two main functions; to counteract the effects of venous hypertension and control oedema. External support will counteract the abnormally high pressure in the superficial veins, emptying them into the deep system and allowing the calf muscle pump to aid the return of the blood to the heart. Compression of the legs may also assist the calf muscle pump by providing a firm 'skin' for the muscles to act against. Their efficacy in increasing the velocity of blood flow in the deep femoral vein (Lawrence and Kakkar, 1980); reducing ambulatory venous pressure (Jones et al, 1980, Horner et al, 1980); reducing oedema (Myers et al, 1972) and relieving symptoms (Somerville et al, 1974) is well established. More recent work has indicated that external compression therapy restores valve function in a proportion of superficial and deep veins by decreasing vein diameter and therefore improving overall venous function (Sarin et al, 1992).

How Much Pressure?

The actual amount of pressure needed to aid venous return and prevent oedema forming is controversial, with proposals ranging from 22 to 40 mmHg. In general terms it is dependent on the severity of the condition (Partsch, 1984; Cornwall et al, 1987). Based on this, a Class II–Class III stocking is the garment of choice although a low pressure is better than no pressure. Struckman (1986) demonstrated that even low pressures increase the effectiveness of the calf muscle pump and that there were reductions in pigmentation, eczema and oedema. Elastic hosiery is capable of exerting pressures of up to 60 mmHg or greater over bony prominences. The Drug Tariff specification grades stockings according to the pressure that they provide at the ankle and regulates the minimum amount of graduation up the leg, as well as stipulating the minimum thickness of yarn to be used in manufacture. There are three classes of stocking, shown in table 8.1. These specifications were implemented in 1988 after the publication of the British Standard for compression hosiery. Stockings are graded into four grades in Europe; Grade 4 giving pressures of over 59 mmHg at the ankle. Grade 4 stockings are only rarely indicated, and are available through some hospital surgical appliance departments. However as

Table 8.1   Compression classes for elastic hosiery

Class 1 gives 14–17 mmHg at the ankle and is for light support. These garments are suitable for
     treating mild varicose veins.

Class 2 gives 18–24 mmHg at the ankle and is for medium support. These garments can be used for
     varicose veins of medium severity; they can be used for treatment and prevention of venous
     ulcers and for mild oedema.

Class 3 gives 25–35 mmHg at the ankle and is for strong support. These garments are used for
     chronic venous insufficiency, severe varicose veins, oedema and the treatment and prevention of
     venous ulcers.

Ruckley stated in 1992 "the pressures specified by the manufacturers on the basis of bench tests seldom reflect the actual pressures measured on the patient's leg".

Graduation

A below-knee compression stocking should exert the greatest pressure at the ankle, progressively decreasing to a lower pressure at the calf; a process known as 'graduated compression'. Using the law of Laplace, a garment that is applied at a constant tension will produce graduated compression, providing it is shaped to fit as accurately at the ankle as at the calf. Pressure varies around the circumference of the leg and will be greatest over bony prominences.

Cornwall et al (1987) studied 15 types of below-knee compression stocking, and found that only five showed satisfactory graduation of pressure. They were able to demonstrate that unsatisfactory pressure gradients correlated with inadequate effects on venous function (measured by photoplethysmography). The technique of photoplethysmography has been described in depth by Cornwall et al elsewhere (1986).

METHODS OF TESTING

Indirect Methods

There are several devices used for indirectly determining stocking pressures. Basically sub-stocking pressures are calculated, using Laplace's Law, for a range of artificially-induced tensions. Unfortunately, compression pressures are measured by different methods in different countries, and the results of the different methods cannot be easily compared. The Hohenstein technique is used in Europe, the Instron method in the United States and the Hatra method in the UK. The Hatra (Hosiery Trades Research Association) device consists of two flat bars arranged to give a simplified leg form. The garment is applied and stretched over the two bars. The tension that develops in the extended garment is measured at set points along its length (ankle, calf and thigh) and this reading is converted to pressure.

Direct Methods

There are a number of devices for determining stocking pressures using the direct method. The Medical Stocking Tester (MST) developed by Borgnis at the Institute of Technology in Zurich has been used internationally. Measurements can be performed whilst the patient is wearing the stocking. The advantage of this method is that the clinician attending the patient can make the measurement in a matter of minutes, thus checking that an individual garment fits and graduates properly.

WHICH TYPE OF STOCKING

There is an enormous variety of compression stockings on the market, and fortunately since the 1988 change in specifications, some of the most effective stockings are available on the FP10 (table 8.2). There are also different types of hosiery, unavailable on FP10, but available through the surgical appliance departments of hospitals. It makes sense to discharge hospital patients where possible, with garments that they can obtain in the community. Dale and Gibson (1989) 'road-tested' a number of the stockings available on prescription for comfort and ease of application. They found that on the whole, compression stockings are comfortable to wear, provided the leg length is correct and that they are properly applied. Open toes and fabrics with a nap were much easier to apply. A number of styles are available including below-knee, thigh-length for use with a suspender belt, thigh length for use with a waist attachment, tights for women and socks of ordinary appearance for men. Unfortunately thigh-length stockings with waist attachment and tights are unavailable on FP10. Stockings may have open or closed toes.

Table 8.2 Graduated compression hosiery available on FP10

Stocking	Manufacturer	Class		
		I	II	III
Lastosheer Sock for men	Kendall Ltd	*	*	
Lastosheer below-knee, thigh-length	Kendall Ltd	*	*	*
Lastoyarn below-knee, thigh-length	Kendall Ltd		*	
Credalast below-knee, thigh-length	Credenhill Ltd	*	*	*
Venosan below-knee, thigh-length	Credenhill Ltd	*	*	*
Duomed below-knee, thigh-length	Medi UK Ltd	*	*	*
Eesilite below-knee, thigh-length	Sallis Ltd	*	*	*
Eesiness Circular below-knee, thigh-length	Sallis Ltd		*	
Eesiness Flatbed below-knee, thigh-length	Sallis Ltd		*	
Nyfine Thigh-Length	Sallis Ltd	*		
Serene Thigh-Length	Sallis Ltd	*		
Mens Support Hose	Scholl Ltd		*	
New Duofine below-knee, thigh-length	Scholl Ltd			*
New Nylastik below-knee, thigh-length	Scholl Ltd	*		
New Sheer Softgrip below-knee, thigh-length	Scholl Ltd		*	
Softgrip below-knee, thigh-length	Scholl Ltd		*	

If stock sizes are not suitable, stockings can be made to measure.

Some patients may be allergic to the elastodiene, rubber, nylon, elastane or lycra that the majority of stockings are manufactured with. A layer of 'tubifast' underneath the stocking may remedy this, but a garment manufactured with a high percentage of cotton should be prescribed for any patient with such an allergy.

The hosiery prescription must specify the class of compression, the desired length (whether thigh-length or below-knee) and the number of pairs to be issued.

If both legs are affected, two pairs of stockings are required; the use of long-term compression is by no means cheap for those who are not exempt from prescription charges.

CORRECT FITTING

Support stockings will not be successful unless they are properly fitted. The vast majority of patients with healed ulcers only require a below-knee support stocking. Compliance is better with below-knee stockings as they are easier to apply, particularly for the elderly. If thigh-length stockings are prescribed, a stocking with a waistband attached should be used, as suspender-supported stockings tend to fall down.

It is important that support hosiery is regarded as an active treatment, and its use appropriately monitored for correct fit, application, patient compliance, comfort and therapeutic effect. In many hospitals, a trained fitter measures the leg and ensures a good fit. In the community, the measurements are usually left to the community or practice nurse. The patient should be standing and the measurements required (in cm) are:

1. The leg circumference at the thinnest part of the ankle.
2. The leg circumference at the fattest part of the calf.
3. The length, measured from the base of the heel to just below the knee.

For full-length stockings, the circumference of the middle of the thigh should also be measured and the length is then measured from the base of the heel to the groin. In the case of the patient who does not fit 'off-the shelf' garments; typically those who have narrow ankles and thin calves or 'champagne-bottle legs', a detailed measurement chart will be supplied by the pharmacist and the stockings made to measure. It is advisable to re-measure the patient when renewing the stockings.

The correct procedure for applying support stockings is shown in figure 8.1. Stockings with an open toe are easier to apply than those with a closed toe. Sprinkling the leg with talcum powder and/or the wearing of fine rubber gloves may aid application, and prevent damage to the stockings from sharp fingernails.

Stockings are not put on like ordinary hosiery. If the stockings are gathered together in the typical 'doughnut' fashion, the effect of the elastic material is multiplied many times and makes application difficult.

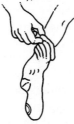

(a.) Insert hand into stocking as far as the heel pocket.

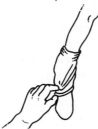

(b.) Grasp centre of heel pocket and turn stocking inside out to heel area.

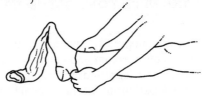

(c.) Carefully position stocking over foot and heel. Be sure the heel is centred in heel pocket.

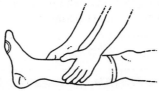

(d.) Pull stocking up and fit around ankle and calf, working up to final position. (Top of stocking is positioned approximately 1-2 inches below bottom of knee cap.)

Fig 8.1   Procedure for applying support stockings

PATIENT COMPLIANCE

Careful explanation of the reasons for and importance of wearing compression hosiery is vital. Support stockings must be worn for life, unless the underlying venous disease has been fully corrected by surgery or sclerotherapy.

At the time of the first prescription it is important to spend time with the patient, explaining the procedure and checking the patient is fully able to apply the garments. Sometimes it is necessary to find a relative or friend who can help an elderly patient to apply their stockings. Although aids to stocking application, such as the Medi Valet, are available, it is often very difficult for the patient to apply the stocking to the aid itself. Ideally, support stockings should be removed at night and re-applied in the morning; however, if this is difficult for a patient to achieve, they can be left *in situ* overnight. A visit to the chiropodist is advisable if hard skin on the feet, rough toenails and/or bunions are causing the stocking to be uncomfortable.

A proportion of patients exhibit an element of self-neglect (Cornwall et al, 1986) and unfortunately there will inevitably be some non-compliance. Ruckley (1992) found that approximately one third of patients do not comply with long-term use of compression hosiery, even with personal supervision from nurses experienced in the care of ulcer patients. If a patient is totally non-compliant with support stockings, an alternative solution is for the patient to wear one or two layers of shaped tubular bandage.

THE NEED FOR FOLLOW-UP

To keep the limb healthy, and hopefully prevent recurrence, it is vital that the patient receives continued encouragement and education. Support stockings should be checked for signs of wear and tear, and new ones prescribed when necessary. It is not always practical for a patient to attend a 'healed-ulcer clinic', particularly if they require transport. Follow-up visits may be more easily arranged via the community nurse or practice nurse. If this is not possible on a regular basis, the patient should be given a contact number and encouraged to get in touch with the nurse or clinic if problems occur. The need to contact the nurse within a day or two if skin breakdown occurs must be impressed upon the patient, as early ulceration is much easier to treat.

WASHING AND LIFESPAN OF ELASTIC STOCKINGS

Frequent washing prolongs the life of a stocking and improves performance by restoring the shape. A choice of washing procedures are laid down by the British Standards Institution, and the manufacturers are required to supply these instructions. Basically, stockings should be washed by hand in warm, soapy water and dried away from direct heat or sunlight. With care, good quality stockings will give adequate pressure after three to four months. They should be replaced according to the manufacturers' instructions, which is usually at 3–6 month intervals.

CONTRA-INDICATIONS OF SUPPORT STOCKINGS

Like many effective treatments, the inappropriate use of compression therapy can cause serious injury. If the leg becomes oedematous, it is important to reduce the oedema by bedrest, or the use of intermittent pneumatic compression therapy (Keachie 1992). I have personally witnessed the top of a stocking causing a band of constriction in an oedematous leg, with subsequent ulceration below the knee.

Foot pulses should be checked each time the stockings are renewed. Limbs with a degree of arterial insufficiency should not be compressed, as this will further impair the blood supply, causing pressure necrosis which may lead to amputation (Callam et al, 1987). Compression stockings should also be used with caution in patients with diabetes mellitus or rheumatoid arthritis. These patients are susceptible to small vessel disease and the application of compression could further occlude these tiny vessels, resulting in pressure necrosis.

SUMMARY

- Leg ulcer recurrence rates are high.
- Expert opinion and some follow-up studies support the notion that the wearing of compression hosiery after ulcer healing helps to reduce ulcer recurrence. There have been no randomized controlled trials to test this.
- Compression hosiery counteracts venous hypertension and controls oedema. The optimum pressure required to achieve this is not known.
- Compression hosiery should not be applied to legs with arterial disease, and should be used with caution in diabetes mellitus and rheumatoid arthritis, due to the risk of small vessel disease.
- Patients should be accurately measured to ensure that compression hosiery fits. The patient's ability to apply the stockings should be evaluated.
- Patients require careful instructions as to the correct application and care of stockings. It is essential to explain the reasons for, and importance of wearing compression hosiery.
- It is important that patients are followed up, where possible, after ulcer healing, in order that skin condition can be monitored and further ulceration spotted and treated early. Follow-up can be achieved through 'healed ulcer clinics' or home visits from community nurses; however, if these are impossible the patient should be given a contact number for use in case of further skin problems or threatened ulceration.

Acknowledgement

Figure 8.1 is reproduced with the kind permission of the Wound Care Society.

References

British Standards Institution (1985) *British Standards Specification for Graduated Compression Hosiery (BS6612)*. London: British Standards Institution.

Browse N L (1983) Venous ulceration. *British Medical Journal*, **286**: 1920–1922.

Callam M J, Ruckley C V, Harper D R and Dale J J (1985) Chronic ulceration of the leg: extent of the problem and provision of care. *British Medical Journal*, **290**: 1855–1856.

Callam M J, Ruckley C V, Dale J J and Harper D R (1987) Hazards of compression treatment of the leg: an estimate from Scottish surgeons. *British Medical Journal*, **295**: 1382.

Cherry G W (1986) Leg ulcers: in support of stockings. *Community Outlook*, **October 8**: 29–31.

Cornwall J V (1985) Diagnosis of leg ulcers. *Journal of District Nursing*, **September**: 4–11.

Cornwall J (1990) Update on leg ulcer survey. *Journal of District Nursing*, **8**(11): 9–10.

Cornwall J V, Dore C J and Lewis J D (1986) Leg ulcers: epidemiology and aetiology. *British Journal of Surgery*, **73**: 693–696.

Cornwall J V, Dore C J and Lewis J D (1987) Graduated compression and its relation to venous refilling time. *British Medical Journal*, **295**: 1087–1090.

Cornwall J V, Dore C J and Lewis J D (1989) Leg ulcers resurrected – a seven year follow-up. Paper presented at *Venous Forum Meeting, Royal Society of Medicine*, May 12.

Dale J J and Gibson B (1989) Which compression stocking? *Professional Nurse*, **July**: 550–556.

Davison A W (1970) *Derby, its Rise and Progress*. Wakefield: SR Publishers.

Dinn E and Henry M (1992) Treatment of venous ulceration by injection sclerotherapy and compression hosiery: a five year study. *Phlebology*, **7**: 23–26.

Horner J, Fernandes J and Fernandes E. (1980) Value of graduated compression stocking in deep venous insufficiency. *British Medical Journal*, **280**: 820–821.

Jones N A G, Webb P J, Rees R I and Kakkar W (1980) A physiological study of elastic compression stockings in venous disorders of the leg. *British Journal of Surgery*, **67**: 569–572.

Keachie J V (1992) *Compression Therapy—A Treatment in its Own Right. Educational Leaflet No. 9*. Northampton: Wound Care Society.

Lawrence D and Kakkar W (1980) Graduated static external compression of the lower limb. *British Journal of Surgery*, **67**: 119–121.

Mayberry J C, Moneta G L, Taylor L M Jr and Porte J M (1991) Fifteen year results of ambulatory compression therapy for chronic venous ulcers. *Surgery*, **109**: 575–581.

Monk B E and Sarkany I (1982) Outcome of treatment of venous stasis ulcers. *Clinical and Experimental Dermatology*, **7**: 397–400.

Myers M B, Rightor M and Cherry G W (1972) Relationship between oedema and the healing rate of stasis ulcers of the leg. *American Journal of Surgery*, **124**: 666–668.

Nash T P (1991) Venous ulceration: factors influencing recurrence after standard surgical problems. *Medical Journal of Australia*, **154**: 48–50.

Partsch H (1984) Do we need firm compression stockings exerting high pressure? *Vasa*, **13**: 52–57.

Ruckley C V (1992) Treatment of venous ulceration – compression therapy. *Phlebology (Suppl)*, **1**: 22–26.

Sarin S, Scurr J H and Coleridge-Smith P D (1992) Mechanism of action of external compression on venous function. *British Journal of Surgery*, **76**: 499–502.

Skene A I, Smith J M, Dore C J, Charlett A and Lewis J D (1992) Venous leg ulcers: a prognostic index to predict time to healing. *British Medical Journal*, **305**: 1119–1121.

Somerville J J I, Brow G O, Byrne P J, Quill R D and Fegan W G (1974) The effect of elastic stockings on superficial venous pressures in patients with venous insufficiency. *British Journal of Surgery*, **64**: 979–981.

Struckman J (1986) Compression stockings and their effect on the venous pump – a comparative study. *Phlebology*, **1**: 37–45.

Wiseman R (1676) *Severall Chirurgicall Treatises*. London: Royson Tooke.

9

Contact Sensitivity and
Eczema in Leg Ulcer Patients

INTRODUCTION

Leg ulcers are an important cause of morbidity, constituting a major problem for the patients who have them and the health care professionals who treat them. The cost to the health service is considerable and was estimated to be in the region of £300–600 million per annum at a Department of Health Seminar in 1989.

A chronic leg ulcer results when there is a failure of the normal healing process, and reflects various underlying problems and pathological conditions. Epidemiological studies by Cornwall et al (1986), Kulozic et al (1986) and Callam et al (1987) have found that approximately 70 per cent of all leg ulcers in the UK are associated with venous insufficiency and chronic venous hypertension. Contact sensitivity is a frequent complication in patients with chronic venous leg ulcers (table 9.1). The management of such patients is difficult, time-consuming and can be extremely costly if the allergens are not identified, and the patient may have several treatments applied in an attempt to avoid the allergen responsible. Although contact sensitivity associated with venous insufficiency has been recognised for many years, results from studies since the 1970s have mainly been published in medical or dermatological journals. Nursing awareness of these articles is likely to be low. There was very little published on this subject in the popular nursing journals until 1990, when Cameron described a study that established the benefits of patch testing, and Cameron and Powell (1992) examined the association between contact dermatitis and non-healing leg ulcers. Callam et al (1985) established that although leg ulcer care was provided by many specialties throughout the health service, the main burden of care fell to the community nurses. Eagle (1990) examined the extent of the problem of leg ulcers nationally and estimated that the changing demography may increase the contribution of leg ulcer management to the community nursing case load. If nurses are to provide the optimum care for their patients, it is essential that they have results of studies made available to them.

This chapter will consider the issue of contact sensitivity in leg ulcer patients, reflect on the results of past and current studies, and consider how these results can influence current practice in the management of leg ulcers.

Table 9.1   Contact sensitivity in leg ulcer patients

Reference	Frequency (%)	Common sensitizers
Malten et al (1973)	76	p-phenylenediamine (PPD), balsam of Peru, benzocaine, wool alcohols, eucerin
Breit (1977)	53.4	benzocaine, neomycin, balsam of Peru, wool alcohols, parabens, gentamicin
Blondeel et al (1978)	85.2	balsam of Peru, wool alcohols, neomycin, cetyl alcohol, parabens, benzocaine
Fraki et al (1979)	69	neomycin, framycetin, wool alcohols, PPD, balsam of Peru
Dooms-Goossens et al (1979)	63	wool alcohols, balsam of Peru, benzocaine, parabens, neomycin
Malten and Kuiper (1985)	69	wool alcohols, fragrance, neomycin, balsam of Peru, eucerin, PPD
Kulozic et al (1988)	51	wool alcohols, neomycin, framycetin, fragrance mix, ester gum resin, gentamicin
Paramsothy et al (1988)	55	wool alcohols, neomycin, fragrance mix, balsam of Peru, parabens, colophony, PPD mix
Cameron (1990)	58	wool alcohols, neomycin, framycetin, parabens, cetylstearyl alcohol, ester gum resin/colophony
Wilson et al (1991)	67	wool alcohols, neomycin, framycetin, gentamicin, cetylstearyl alcohol

ECZEMA

Leg ulcers present as moist, open wounds; often with surrounding stasis eczema (plate 22). In such patients, the eczema may be related to venous stasis or may be a contact dermatitis which may be irritant or allergic or a combination of both. Eczema, also referred to as 'dermatitis' presents as an itchy, inflammatory condition of the skin; characterised by erythema, weeping and scaling.

There are two types of eczema:

● **Endogenous eczema**—related to constitutional (internal) factors.
● **Exogenous eczema**—related to contact with external substances.

VENOUS STASIS (VARICOSE) ECZEMA

Venous stasis eczema is endogenous and commences on the inner aspect of the lower leg, just above the area of the medial malleolus. Skin changes occur in patients with chronic venous hypertension due to the leaking of haemosiderin from the red blood cells, through the capillaries into the interstitial space. This may be seen clinically as a brownish staining of the skin, particularly in the area above the medial malleolus, and is a condition described by Burnand et al (1982) as **lipodermatosclerosis**. The latter group also showed that this condition was associated with fibrin cuff formation around the capillaries, possibly leading to impaired tissue oxygenation. Coincident to these findings is the onset of venous stasis eczema, although it is unclear why poor tissue perfusion and high venous pressure causes eczema.

CONTACT DERMATITIS

Contact dermatitis is an exogenous eczema, and may be due to irritants or allergens.

Irritant Contact Dermatitis

The application of irritants to the skin around a leg ulcer, or to skin demonstrating a stasis eczema, or exudate leaking from a leg ulcer on to the surrounding skin, may lead to the development of an irritant contact dermatitis. This may act in a similar way to an allergic contact dermatitis to increase morbidity and delay healing.

Substances that can cause an irritant contact dermatitis are sometimes used in the treatment of leg ulcers, and include antiseptics, some medicaments and moisturisers, and bandages applied directly to the skin.

Allergic Contact Dermatitis

Baer (1986) describes the occurrence of contact dermatitis as the result of cell-mediated, delayed hypersensitivity, induced by the reaction between a specific antigen and immunologically competent lymphocytes. This may be seen as a defence reaction of the body against topical sensitisers (allergens), which have come into contact with the skin.

Bahmer (1989) suggests that the frequent application of topical therapies for a prolonged contact time to antigen-presenting cells, results in the development of sensitivity to the allergen. On further exposure, the skin develops an eczematous reaction—an allergic, contact dermatitis.

Sensitization may occur after short exposure to an allergen of 10–14 days or even after several years of using a substance where no previous problems have occurred. The eczema will show in the area of direct contact with the allergen. If the reaction is severe there could be a secondary spread, where the eczematous reaction extends beyond the area of direct contact and can include other parts of the body such as the arms or trunk.

To prevent or identify a contact sensitivity, patch testing can be undertaken using standard commercially-available materials.

PATCH TESTING

Indications for patch testing patients with leg ulceration are:

● Presence of eczema around a leg ulcer.
● An ulcer that should heal, but is failing to do so.
● History of a reaction to topical treatment.

Patch testing is a scientific method of investigation, with a defined code of practice and methodology that requires referral to a dermatologist. The International Contact Dermatitis Research Group (ICDRG) guidelines recommended by Wilkinson et al (1970), determine the concentrations and suggest suitable vehicles for the purpose of patch testing. A set of allergens grouped together is referred to as a 'battery', e.g. the European Standard Battery (table 9.2). The ICDRG also define the guidelines for reading and interpreting the patch test results. Studies between different centres can be compared if they have adhered to the standards set up by the ICDRG.

Table 9.2   Oxfordshire Area Health Authority (Department of Dermatology): European Standard Battery

Allergen	Present in
Potassium dichromate	cement, chrome, tanned leather
Nickel sulphate	metal alloys, jewellery, e.g. ear rings, clothes, e.g. bra clips, jeans studs
Cobalt chloride	cement, metal alloys, pigment in paint
Thiuram mix	accelerator in rubber and other industrial use
Mercapto mix	accelerator in rubber and other industrial use
Mercaptobenzothiazole	accelerator in rubber and other industrial use
Black rubber mix	black rubbers, e.g. tyres
Neomycin sulphate	antibiotic
Benzocaine	topical local anaesthetic (insect bite creams and creams for piles).
Quinoline mix	antibacterial agents in creams and bandages
Epoxy resin	Two-part glues, e.g. Araldite
4-tert-butylphenol formaldehyde resin	adhesive used in shoes
4-phenylenediamine base (PPD)	hairdyes
Colophony	sticking plaster, oils, fluxes
Parabens mix	preservatives in creams (cosmetic and medicament)
Wool alcohols	creams, ointments, cosmetics, hand lotions
Ethylenediamine dihydrochloride	preservative in Tri-Adcortyl cream
Quaternium 15 (Dowicil 200)	preservative in cosmetics
CI + Me Isothiazolinone (Kathon CG)	preservative in cosmetics
Formaldehyde	preservative-cosmetics, cleansers, detergents; clothing as anti-crease preparation
Balsam of Peru	perfumes, make up, medicaments
Fragrance mix	perfumes
Primin	primula plant
Sesquiterpene lactone mix	plants—compositae

Leg ulcer patients are patch tested to the European Standard Battery (which contains the most frequently encountered environmental allergens, many of which are of relevance to leg ulcer patients) and a battery of allergens relative to their specific treatment.

Finn chambers (Epitest Ltd, Oy, Finland) on Scanpor surgical tape (Norgest plaster, Oslo, Norway) are filled with small amounts of the test substances. The prepared test strips are then applied to normal skin on the patient's upper back (day 1) (plate 23). Active dermatitis should not be present at the time of patch testing. If any eczema is present, this should be treated before the patch tests are applied. The locations of the test chambers are marked on the patient's skin using a suitable skin marker. After 2 days (on day 3), the test strips are removed and the skin on the back allowed to settle for a period of 30 minutes, before the first reading is recorded. A further reading is taken 2 days later (day 5).

Paramsothy et al (1988) confirmed this combination of days as being the most accurate for the reading of patch tests. The extent of erythema, eczema, oedematous and vesicular involvement is recorded at each reading. A positive reaction is defined as the presence of erythema and vesiculation (eczema) at the test site (plate 24). Some allergens are late reactors and a further reading may occasionally be required.

Negative Patch Testing

In patients with a leg ulcer and eczema, extensive patch testing may sometimes produce a negative result. This may be due to a missed allergen, use of oral or topical corticosteroids (which suppress the inflammatory response), or may mean that the eczema is an irritant contact dermatitis or a stasis eczema.

LEG ULCER ALLERGENS (SEE TABLE 9.3)

Lanolin

Tested as **wool alcohols, amerchol** and **eucerin**. Sensitivity to lanolin has been recognised for many years in patients with stasis dermatitis and leg ulcers. Lanolin is still widely used as an emollient and moisturiser and further cases of sensitivity continue to occur (table 9.1). Whether these patients have a new sensitivity or a long-standing sensitivity newly recognised is unclear. Products containing lanolin should not be used on patients with leg ulcers.

Topical Antibiotics

Allergy to topical antibiotics remains a problem with **neomycin, framycetin** and **gentamicin** being the most common sensitizers. They are all aminoglycoside antibiotics and a positive reaction to one of the group means that they should all be avoided. Neomycin is a late reactor, and a further reading may be necessary 10 days after the application of the patch test. The use of topical antibiotics can lead to the emergence of multi-resistant organisms as well as sensitivity and should be avoided (*British Medical Journal*, 1977).

Perfumes

Balsam of Peru and **Fragrance mix** are related to perfume sensitivity. Perfumes are found in many over-the-counter moisturisers, including many baby preparations. Patients should be encouraged to use a simple emollient, such as white soft paraffin.

Preservatives and Biocides

Parabens. The preservatives within paste bandages and other topical preparations may sensitise. The parabens group has been found to be a common sensitizer in leg ulcer patients. It is present in some creams and paste bandages. Health care professionals need to be aware of changes in the formulation of paste bandages. A list of ingredients is usually included in the packaging of a paste bandage and the alternative preservatives used in place of parabens may also sensitise, e.g. **phenosept** in Calaband™ paste bandage (Seton).

   Quinoline mix (3 per cent clioquinol/3 per cent chlorquinadiol) is sometimes used as an antimicrobial. Clioquinol is present in Quinaband™ paste bandage (Seton).

   Chloroxylenol is a common antiseptic, present in Dettol, which many elderly people have put into their baths for years. It is sometimes used elsewhere as a preservative.

   Chlorhexidine. Although chlorhexidine, present in Bactigras™ (Smith & Nephew), has been reported as a significant sensitiser in a Danish study (Knudsen and Avnstorp, 1991), it has not been shown to be a common sensitizer in the UK.

Vehicle

Cetylstearyl alcohol. This is an important allergen that is particularly difficult to avoid as it is present in many topical cream preparations, moisturisers and emollients and some paste bandages.

Rubber

Mercapto/thiuram mix/carba mix are accelerators used in the manufacture of rubber. Rubber is present in many elastic bandages and elastic tubular bandage such as Tubigrip™ (Seton). Protecting the skin first, with gauze or cotton tubular bandage helps to prevent the rubber from coming into contact with the skin.

Adhesive

Colophony/ester gum resin is found in the adhesive backing of tapes and some bandages. Tapes should never be applied directly to the skin on a patient with a leg ulcer or eczematous skin. Likewise, the adhesive backing on bandages should never be allowed to touch the skin.

Local Anaesthetic

Benzocaine was a common sensitizer in the 1970s. It is present in over-the-counter preparations used to reduce irritation and for the treatment of haemorrhoids.

Dyes

The allergen *p*-phenylenediamine **(PPD)** has gradually lost its importance over the years. Malten and Kuiper (1985) reported that the early high numbers of allergies were attributed to the fact that bandages were dyed, and numbers reduced as white bandages became popular and dyeing techniques improved.

Table 9.3 Oxford Department of Dermatology (Churchill Hospital): leg ulcer allergens

Allergens	Sources
Lanolin	
wool alcohols	Many creams, ointments, emollients and moisturisers, e.g. E45 cream,
amerchol	Oilatum, Hydrous ointment
eucerin	
Topical antibiotics	Found in many medicaments:
Framycetin	Sofratulle
Neomycin	Cicatrin powder and some other medicaments
Gentamicin	Gentamicin cream and ointment
Preservatives and biocides	In some medicaments and paste bandages:
Parabens	Icthaband, Zincaband, Viscopaste PB7 paste bandages
Phenosept	Calaband paste bandage
Chloroxynenol	Dettol
Quinoline mix	Antiseptics and Quinaband paste bandage
Vehicles	Present in cream preparations, e.g.
Cetyl alcohol	Hioxyl, Flamazine, E45, Aqueous cream, Corticosteroid creams
Stearyl alcohol	also present in emulsifying ointment and Icthopaste and
Cetylstearyl alcohol	Vicopaste PB7 bandages
Adhesives	
Ester gum resin	Sticking plaster, adhesive on back of some bandages
Colophony	Cohesive bandages
Rubber mixes	
Thiuram	
Mercapto	Elastic tubular bandages, some bandages and elastic stockings
Carba	
Perfume	
Balsam of Peru	In some medicaments, baby preparations and bath additives
Fragrance Mix	

STUDIES OF CONTACT SENSITIVITY

Allergy to components of topical preparations is common in patients with leg ulcers. Studies by Blondeel et al (1978) and Dooms-Goossens et al (1979) have suggested that the prevalence of contact sensitivity is between two and five times higher in leg ulcer patients than the general background population in a dermatology clinic. The incidence is further increased if the patients have co-existing eczema; a common complication in leg ulcer patients. Paramsothy et al (1988) found 47 per cent of patients tested had eczema around the ulcer, characterised by itching, vesiculation and exudation or past evidence of these. Results showed that these patients were more likely to have positive patch test results than patients without surrounding eczema. Kulozic et al (1988) looked specifically at community-based patients, and found allergic reactions occurred in 50.8 per cent of patients and were significantly higher in patients with co-existing eczema. Paramsothy et al (1988) found an association between the duration of the ulcer and the number of contact sensitivities. A review of the incidence of contact sensitivity in patients with stasis dermatitis between 1972 and 1977 by Breit (1977) showed an average of 62.5 per cent. The most common sensitizers were reported to be wool alcohols, neomycin, parabens and Balsam of Peru.

Recently Wilson et al (1991) reported that contact sensitivity remains a considerable problem with 67 per cent of patients developing an allergic reaction. The most common sensitizers were reported to be wool alcohols, neomycin, framycetin, gentamicin and cetylstearyl alcohol.

Although the incidence of contact sensitivity remains much the same, there has been some change in the distribution of the allergens (table 9.1). This could reflect changing practices in leg ulcer management.

PATCH TEST RESULTS IN CLINICAL PRACTICE

Following patch testing, it is essential that the results are well documented in the patient's notes and care plans, so that allergens that have been shown to be sensitisers can be avoided in treatment. Local contact dermatitis can cause irritation and discomfort to the patient. Scratching of the affected area can result in superficial erosions. If left untreated, the erosions could extend beyond the depths of the epidermis, resulting in extension of the existing ulcerated areas or the development of new ulcerated areas. Identification of the allergen and a subsequent change in treatment can sometimes result in the healing of the leg ulcer.

Identification of allergens is a problem in the UK as manufacturers are not required to list the ingredients of their products on the packaging and the information provided varies considerably. Some products on the market have all the ingredients listed, some have only a few of the ingredients listed, and some even state what the product *does not* contain, without giving any information as to its actual contents! Where patients have been shown to be sensitised to the constituents of topical agents commonly used in the treatment of leg ulcers, a change in treatment could re-expose the patient to the allergen, as it may be present in several different medicaments. It is therefore essential that information regarding possible sources of the allergen is given to both the Primary Health Care Team and the patient. A handout listing potential leg ulcer allergens, and the products in which they are contained, is given to patients and their professional carers following patch testing at the Oxford Dermatology Clinic (table 9.3). Identification of contact sensitivities can reduce the morbidity related to a contact dermatitis, allowing treatment to be planned with confidence on a rational and therefore cost-effective basis.

The company should be contacted directly for information and advice if there is any doubt as to whether a product is suitable for a patient with a known allergy. Any information acquired should be well documented in the patient's notes.

MANAGEMENT OF CONTACT DERMATITIS

Many topical applications are used in the treatment of leg ulcers, including primary ulcer dressings, applications to the surrounding skin and various bandages. Applications are often applied for long periods of time, under occlusion and on eczematous skin. Even when common sensitisers are avoided, patients with leg ulcers may still become allergic to any part of their treatment. In some instances these may be isolated cases. There have been reactions to Flamazine™ (Smith and Nephew) reported by Rasmussen (1984) and Paramsothy et al (1988), and Hyoxil™ (Quinoderm) reported by Wilson et al (1991). Recently, Mallon and Powell (1993) reported on two patients sensitized to Granuflex E™ (now known as new improved formulation Granuflex (ConvaTec) and even simple non-adherent dressings have been reported by Duhra and Charles-Holmes (1992) to have sensitised one patient.

IRRITANT CONTACT DERMATITIS

Protection of the surrounding skin, particularly that distal to the ulcer, is extremely important. Cherry et al (1991) have found zinc oxide paste to be effective in protecting this vulnerable area from wound exudate. Antiseptics should be avoided and bandages should never be applied directly to the skin.

ACUTE ECZEMA

An acute eczema will require treatment with a topical corticosteroid preparation. The potency needed will depend on the severity of the eczema. The use of corticosteroid ointments that are in a white soft paraffin base, are less likely to cause problems than cream preparations containing cetylstearyl alcohol. Topical steroids may occasionally induce allergy, as reported by Hannuksela and Salo (1986), seen as contact dermatitis or a poor response to treatment. The frequency of application of a topical steroid ointment may be daily at first, or at each dressing change. The frequency should be reduced slowly, and the steroid ointment gradually replaced with a simple emollient such as 50 per cent white soft paraffin/50 per cent liquid paraffin. Moisturisers containing cetylstearyl alcohol should be avoided (table 9.3).

The development of an acute eczema in a patient who has been previously patch tested and allergen exposure eliminated is an indication for repeat patch testing, as new allergens may have developed. Secondary infection is a complication of eczema that requires treatment with a systemic antibiotic.

VENOUS STASIS (VARICOSE) ECZEMA

This condition can be improved by elevation of the legs and compression bandaging from toe to knee. A paste bandage containing icthammol is particularly useful to treat the eczema, and patients find the paste bandage cooling to the skin. Dry, scaly skin can be improved by use of a 50 per cent white soft paraffin/50 per cent liquid paraffin emollient. If severe, the eczema can be treated with a corticosteroid ointment as in an acute eczema.

PREVENTION OF CONTACT SENSITIVITY

If nurses are to provide the optimum care for their patients, they need to know what the most common allergens are, where they are to be found, and how they can avoid them in treatment (table 9.3).

A useful plan of management, which aims to avoid irritants and possible allergens, is to:

- Irrigate the ulcer with normal saline.
- Use zinc oxide paste to protect the surrounding skin from wound exudate.
- Use a simple, cost-effective emollient such as white soft paraffin and liquid paraffin, in a 50/50 mixture (this is unlikely to sensitise).
- Use a layer of gauze or tubular cotton bandage or similar, under elastic and adhesive bandages to prevent direct contact with the skin.

Many patients treat themselves with over-the-counter emollients and moisturisers at home, and this must be taken into consideration. Many of these over-the-counter products contain common sensitisers such as lanolin and perfume. Advice to the patient on preparations that are unlikely to sensitise is essential for their subsequent management.

HEALED PATIENTS

Following healing of a venous ulcer, patients should be fitted with a graduated compression stocking. This has been shown by Lewis et al (1976) to increase the velocity of venous blood flow in the legs and lead to a more rapid clearance of stagnant blood from behind venous valves. Struckmann (1986) identified that with continued daytime wear of compression hosiery, there is a reduction in skin pigmentation and eczema. If a patient has an allergic reaction to the compression hosiery it may be due to rubber sensitivity. There are graduated compression stockings available which do not contain rubber and these should be made available to the patient.

SUMMARY

Contact dermatitis is a complicating factor in patients with chronic venous leg ulcers. Kulozic et al (1988) emphasised the importance of early patch testing of leg ulcer patients as an important factor in their management. All patients with long-standing leg ulcers that are failing to heal (despite appropriate treatment), and those with surrounding eczema would benefit from patch testing. Studies have shown that many patch tested patients have multiple positive reactions, complicating local therapy considerably. Without the benefits of patch testing, simply changing the medicament may not be effective, as the same allergen may be present in several different topical applications and medicaments.

Leg ulcer management requires a team approach to care. Dermatologists are an important part of the team who are very willing to help and advise on contact sensitivity. Referral to a dermatologist for patch testing and identification of any contact sensitivities could reduce the morbidity related to its complications. Treatment could be planned and implemented with confidence and relevant changes made on a rational basis. This would increase patient comfort, reduce nursing time and promote more cost-effective practice.

References

Baer R L (1986) The mechanism of allergic contact hypersensitivity. In: *Contact Dermatitis*, 3rd ed, ed. Fisher A A. Philadelphia: Lea & Febiger.

Bahmer F A (1989) Local factors that might promote the development of contact allergies in patients with chronic venous insufficiency. In: *Phlebologie*, eds Davy A and Stemmer R, pp. 110–112. London: Libbey.

Blondeel A, Oleffe J and Achten G (1978) Contact allergy in 330 dermatological patients. *Contact Dermatitis*, **4**: 270–276.

Breit R (1977) Allergen change in stasis dermatitis. *Contact Dermatitis*, **3**: 309–311.

British Medical Journal (1977) Topical antibiotics. *British Medical Journal*, **1**: 1494.

Burnand K G, Whimster I and Naidoo A (1982) Pericapillary fibrin in the ulcer-bearing skin of the leg: the cause of lipodermatosclerosis and venous ulceration. *British Medical Journal* **285**: 1920–1922.

Callam M J, Harper D R, Dale J J and Ruckley C V (1987) Chronic ulcer of the leg: clinical history. *British Medical Journal*, **294**: 1389–91.

Callam M J, Ruckley C V, Harper D R and Dale J J (1985) Chronic ulceration of the leg: extent of the problem and provision of care. *British Medical Journal*, **290**: 1855–1856.

Cameron J (1990) Patch testing for leg ulcers. *Nursing Times*, **86**(25): 63–64.

Cameron J and Powell S (1992) Contact dermatitis: its importance in leg ulcer patients. *Wound Management*, **2**(3): 12–13.

Cherry G W, Cameron J and Ryan T J (1991) *Leg Ulcer Blueprint*. London: ConvaTec Ltd.

Cornwall J V, Dore C and Lewis J (1986) Leg ulcers: epidemiology and aetiology. *British Journal of Surgery*, **73**: 693–696.

Department of Health Seminar (1989) *Gravitational (varicose) Ulcers: The Problem, What We Know and What We Need to Know and Do!* London: Department of Health.

Dooms-Goossens A, Degreef H, Parijs M and Kerkhofs L (1979) A retrospective study of patch test results from 163 patients with stasis dermatitis or leg ulcers. *Dermatologica*, **159**: 93–100.

Duhra P and Charles-Holmes R (1992) Contact sensitivity to NA dressing. *Contact Dermatitis*, **27**: 255–280.

Eagle M (1990) The quiet epidemic below the knee. *Nursing Standard*, **4**(15): 32–36.

Fraki J E, Peltonen L and Hopsu-Havu V K (1979) Allergy to various components of topical preparations in stasis dermatitis and leg ulcer. *Contact Dermatitis*, **5**: 97–100.

Hannuksela M and Salo H (1986) The repeated open application test (ROAT). *Contact Dermatitis*, **14**: 221–227.

Knudsen B B and Avnstorp C (1991) Chlorhexidine gluconate and acetate in patch testing. *Contact Dermatitis*, **24**: 45–49.

Kulozic M, Cherry G W and Ryan T J (1986) The importance of measuring the ankle: brachial systolic pressure ratio in the management of leg ulcers. *British Journal of Dermatology*, **115** Suppl 30: 26–27.

Kulozic M, Powell S M, Cherry G, Ryan T J (1988) Contact Sensitivity in Community-based leg ulcer patients. *Clinical and Experimental Dermatology* **13**: 82–84.

Lewis E L, Antoine J, Mueller C, Talbot W A, Swaroop R and Sterling Edwards W (1976) Elastic compression in the prevention of venous stasis. *American Journal of Surgery*, **132**: 739–743.

Mallon E and Powell S (1993) Contact sensitivity to Granuflex E hydrocolloid dressing. Paper presented at the *British Association of Dermatology Conference*, Oxford, England.

Malten K E, Kuiper J P and van der Staak W B J M (1973) Contact allergic investigations in 100 patients with Ulcus Crurus. *Dermatologica*, **147**: 241–254.

Malten K E and Kuiper J P (1985) Reactions allergiques au contact sur 100 patients selectionnes atteints d'un ulcere de la jambe. *Phlebologie*, **38**: 375–381.

Paramsothy Y, Collins M and Smith A G (1988) Contact dermatitis in patients with leg ulcers. *Contact Dermatitis*, **18**: 30–36.

Rasmussen I (1984) Patch test reactions to Flamazine. *Contact Dermatitis*, **11**: 117.

Struckmann J (1986) Low compression gradient stockings in patients with venous insufficiency: effect on the musculo-venous pump, evaluated by strain gauge plethysmograph. *Phlebology*, **3/4**: 189–196.

Wilkinson D S, Fregert S, Magnusson B, Bandmann H J, Calnan C D, Cronin E, Hjorth N, Maibach H J, Malten K E, Meneghini C L and Pirila V (1970) Terminology of contact dermatitis. *Acta Dermatovener (Stockholm)*, **50**: 287–292.

Wilson C L, Cameron J, Powell S M, Cherry G and Ryan T J (1991) High incidence of contact dermatitis in leg ulcer patients—implications for management. *Clinical and Experimental Dermatology*, **16**: 250–253.

10

The Management of Leg

Ulcers: Current Nursing

Practice

INTRODUCTION

The majority of people with leg ulcers are cared for in the community by nurses (Callam et al, 1985, Cornwall et al, 1986). This chapter examines current nursing practice in leg ulcer management and makes recommendations for its future development.

REVIEW OF KEY RESEARCH

The Lothian and Forth Valley leg ulcer prevalence study, commenced in 1981, reported 1477 patients suffering from chronic leg ulceration, against a background population of approximately 1 million. Five per cent of these individuals were treated as hospital inpatients, 12 per cent were managed jointly between out-patients departments and the primary health care team, and 83 were managed solely in the community, mainly by community nurses (Callam et al, 1985). Other studies report similar figures (e.g. Cornwall et al, 1986, Mallett and Charles, 1990), and despite the recent growth and development of practice nursing and the increased availability of practice nurses in general practice, the majority of patients with leg ulcers are still treated at home by a district nurse (Cullum and Last, 1993). The scope of clinical responsibility of the nurse managing a leg ulcer patient often extends to treatment choice (Ertl, 1992) and it is imperative that the care provided by community nurses has been demonstrated to be both effective and efficient.

Cullum and Last (1993) in their survey of leg ulcer management in the Wirral found that the initial diagnosis of a patient's ulcer was undertaken by a consultant in 28 per cent of cases, by a general practitioner in 48 per cent and by nurses in 19 per cent of cases (*n*=301). Cullum (1994) is concerned that not all patients with leg ulcers are given the benefit of a medical examination and that a medical diagnosis may be attributed by nursing staff with little or no specialist training. To reduce the risk of inappropriate treatment and to maximise the benefit for patients, it is essential that community nurses are adequately trained to undertake the comprehensive nursing assessment of patients with leg ulcers and know when to refer to the GP or hospital consultant.

THE NURSING ASSESSMENT

Browse et al (1988) outline the comprehensive medical assessment of a patient with a leg ulcer and much of this is also pertinent to the nursing assessment. A survey was undertaken by the *Journal of District Nursing* in 1986 wherein readers were asked to complete a questionnaire relating to their management of leg ulcers (*Journal of District Nursing*, 1986). A total of 474 nurses responded to this survey, representing a low response rate, probably biased in favour of those nurses interested in leg ulcers. Respondents were predominantly from the South East of England and based in rural practices. Nurses were asked what they looked for as an indicator of venous disease during their assessment. An assessment of skin colour was included by 77 per cent of nurses; however, only 16 per cent mentioned varicose veins and 10 per cent varicose eczema.

More recently, Roe et al (1993) surveyed the reported nursing practice of 146 community nurses from three district health authorities/community trusts in Mersey Region. Information collected related to the assessment and treatment of patients with leg ulcers, along with advice given regarding prevention of re-ulcer-ation. All data were analysed according to each nurse's year of qualification as a community nurse and their location of work. The syllabus for district nursing underwent a substantial revision from 1981, when the academic content and length of course increased (Panel of Assessors for District Nurse Training, 1976). It was clear that the year a community nurse qualified had an important effect on nurses' reported clinical practice, their continuing education and other related professional issues (Roe and Luker, 1992). The majority of community nurses (n=126; 86 per cent), reported that most of the leg ulcer patients in their care had venous ulcers, whilst fewer nurses (n=62; 42 per cent) cared for people with arterial ulcers; this finding is consistent with epidemiological studies (Callam et al, 1985; Cornwall et al, 1986).

Regarding nursing assessment, 107 (74 per cent) nurses in the Mersey study stated they would obtain information relating to the patient's lifestyle, and included details of their weight, diet, exercise and smoking habits. More nurses who qualified after 1981 (n=65; 76 per cent) obtained information relating to a patient's past medical and surgical history than nurses who qualified before 1981 (n=34; 57 per cent) (P=0.01) (table 10.1). When assessing the general appearance of the leg, 113 (78 per cent), nurses said they would look for oedema, varicose veins and take into account the overall shape of the leg. More nurses (n=120; 83 per cent) looked at the skin condition and made observations about the colour, temperature, presence or absence of hair and eczema, and 115 (79 per cent) nurses would take foot pulses with or without the use of Doppler ultrasound. The taking of foot pulses is one way of assessing whether the leg is receiving a reasonable arterial

Table 10.1 Assessment of medical history by community nurses according to year of qualification

Year of qualification	Assess medical history		Total
	Yes	No	
Up to 1981	34	26	60
1982 onwards	65	20	85
Total	99	46	145

χ^2=6.37; d.f.=1; P=0.01.

inflow (Browse et al 1988). Nurses who qualified after 1981 were more likely (n=76; 89 per cent) to check for pedal pulses than nurses who qualified before 1981 (n=38; 63 per cent) ($P<0.01$) (table 10.2).

Table 10.2 Palpation of pedal pulses by community nurses according to year of qualification

Year of qualification	Palpate pedal pulses		Total
	Yes	No	
Up to 1981	38	22	60
1982 onwards	76	9	85
Total	114	31	145

χ^2=14.23; d.f.=1; $P<0.01$.

Only 35 per cent of nurses who participated in the *Journal of District Nursing* survey included patient's pain in their assessment (*Journal of District Nursing*, 1986). Patient's experience of pain was also poorly assessed in the Roe et al (1993) study, where slightly more than half of the community nurses (n=80; 55 per cent) did not report that they would undertake an assessment of a patient's experience of pain. Of those nurses who did assess the patient's experience of pain, more of them had qualified since 1981 (n=44; 52 per cent), than before 1981 (n=21; 35 per cent) (95 per cent confidence interval from 1 to 33 per cent; P=0.05) (table 10.3). An assessment of pain is an essential feature of any nursing assessment, but particularly so for patients experiencing a painful, chronic condition.

Table 10.3 Assessment of leg ulcer pain by community nurses according to year of qualification

Year of qualification	Assess pain		Total
	Yes	No	
Up to 1981	21	39	60
1982 onwards	44	41	85
Total	65	80	145

χ^2=4.00; d.f.=1; P=0.05.

Less than half the nurses in the Mersey study (n=67; 46 per cent) said they would measure the leg ulcer as part of their initial assessment, although more of them (n=107; 71 per cent) said that they would use measurement as a way of monitoring the ulcer's progress. Obviously, measurement of the ulcer is an important aspect of both assessment and evaluation of progress. Fortunately, grids and acetates for tracing ulcers are supplied with some of the modern wound dressings, which means recording this information can now be more readily carried out.

THE ROLE OF THE NURSE IN TREATMENT CHOICE

The study by Cullum and Last (1993) of the nursing management of leg ulcers in Wirral, Merseyside, examined the origin of current treatment choices for those patients with a leg ulcer during the month of September 1991. Wound dressings were chosen by medical personnel in 44 per cent of cases and by nurses in 53 per cent; bandages were chosen by doctors in 34 per cent of cases and by nurses in 59 per cent. Ertl (1992) found that nurses were wholly responsible for all treatment decisions in 71 per cent of cases. Obviously, community nurses have to make key decisions regarding which wound cleansers, dressings and bandages they use, even if it is the general practitioner who writes out the prescription.

WOUND CLEANSERS

Over zealous cleaning of the leg ulcer may damage newly formed granulation tissue and reduce wound temperature, so delaying healing (Thomas, 1990). Historically, antiseptics were widely used as cleansing agents in an attempt to remove any bacteria from an ulcer. Nowadays it is understood that all ulcers contain commensal organisms, although the effect, if any, of bacteria on wound healing is unclear (Gilchrist, 1989). Using antiseptics such as cetrimide or caustic substances such as hypochlorite as cleansing agents is possibly hazardous and they should not be used (Leaper, 1986, Thomas, 1990). Cleansing the ulcer with warmed saline is the safest option and there is no evidence that complete immersion of the leg in warm water does any harm; indeed it may be psychologically beneficial for patients to have their limbs bathed and may also improve the local circulation and benefit the skin. In the Mersey Region survey (Roe et al, 1994), the majority of nurses (n=110; 75 per cent) said they would bathe patients' legs sometimes, although 32 (22 per cent) community nurses stated they would never immerse an ulcerated leg in water. Not all nurses would use discretion; 74 (53 per cent) of them would routinely cleanse leg ulcers. Fortunately, 115 (79 per cent) nurses reported that they would not use hypochlorite solutions such as Eusol and 94 (64 per cent) would never use cetrimide; in keeping with good practice. Hydrogen peroxide was used by eight nurses within one health authority; this practice is generally not recommended as there have been isolated, although unsubstantiated, reports of risks of fatal air emboli when hydrogen peroxide is used in deep cavity wounds (Sleigh and Winter, 1985). More nurses (56) from one health authority used potassium permanganate as a cleansing solution; this may have been on the basis of a consultant's instructions (Roe et al, 1994); however, there is no evidence to suggest that potassium permanganate makes any useful contribution to the management of patients with leg ulcers.

DRESSINGS

The range of modern wound dressings available on the Drug Tariff (FP10) and used in the community has increased in recent years. Most community nurses have incorporated modern wound dressings in their treatment regimens. In the Mersey study, 133 (91 per cent) community nurses reported that they used hydrocolloids, 127 (87 per cent) alginates, 81 (55 per cent) hydrogels and 98 (67 per cent) polysaccharide beads (Roe et al, 1994), although within this study it was not possible to comment on the appropriateness of usage. Allergies to leg ulcer products are fairly common (Cameron, 1990 and chapter 9); however, not all nurses are aware of this. Only 65 (45 per cent) nurses in the Mersey study knew that the primary dressing could cause an allergic reaction (Roe et al, 1994).

The use of topical antibiotics (available in ointments, creams and tulle dressings) presents problems on two fronts: skin sensitivity to topical antibiotics is common and bacteria can also become resistant to topically applied antibiotics during treatment (*British Medical Journal*, 1977). In the Mersey survey, only four nurses recognised that topical antibiotics could cause an allergic reaction, and only 54 (37 per cent) nurses stated they would not use an antibiotic tulle and 30 (26 per cent) would not use an antibiotic cream. However, the more recently qualified nurses were less likely to use antibiotic tulle or creams than nurses who qualified before 1981 (Roe et al, 1994). In this study it was also found that the majority of nurses (*n*=128; 89 per cent) often used a variety of dressing products in combination, layering a number of primary dressings on top of each other. Such practice is probably wasteful, with no demonstrated therapeutic value. The variety and combination of leg ulcer treatments should be kept simple and to a minimum due to the risk of allergies as well for reasons of economics. Only a minority of nurses (*n*= 21; 14 per cent) stated they would change a dressing as infrequently as possible.

It would appear that the development of research-based management guidelines, by members of the primary health care team, is required in order to rationalise leg ulcer care. This type of practice development offers a means of integrating research findings into practice, thereby improving the quality of patient care and potentially saving money.

BANDAGES

Compression bandaging is the most important aspect of the management of patients with venous ulcers (Blair et al, 1988, Browse et al, 1988) and yet there is evidence that many patients with venous ulceration forgo this part of the treatment. In their 1991 survey of leg ulcer management in Wirral, Merseyside, Cullum and Last (1993) found that only 30 out of a total of 137 leg ulcer patients described as having purely venous ulceration were receiving bandages capable of delivering compression. Crepe bandage and 'straight' (rather than shaped) tubular bandage were the bandages most often worn by patients with venous ulcers in this study, and neither bandage is capable of supplying adequate compression (Thomas, 1990). Fortunately none of the 18 patients described as having purely arterial ulcers was receiving compression.

In the Mersey region survey, only 93 (64 per cent) of community nurses reported that they would apply compression bandaging exclusively to venous ulcers; the remainder applying compression bandages to all other types of ulcer (Roe et al, 1994). The application of compression to legs with substantial arterial disease or to the limbs of patients with diseases such as rheumatoid arthritis or diabetes who may have small vessel disease or vasculitis may be extremely hazardous. In the same study only a minority of nurses (n=33; 23 per cent) had an understanding of the type of bandages capable of achieving a therapeutic level of compression, and only six nurses described an appropriate bandaging technique. A potential for financial savings was once again apparent, as 124 (85 per cent) nurses used multiple bandage systems although only 40 nurses described a combination of bandages deemed suitable (by Thomas, 1990) for the purpose of delivering graduated compression. The use of ineffective bandage systems is obviously wasteful. Again, the development of management guidelines may help to rationalise the use of bandages as a treatment modality for patients with leg ulceration.

ADVICE TO PATIENTS

The community nurse is an important source of advice and information for patients. The information given to patients with venous leg ulcers would be expected to include advice about ways in which the patient may help to promote healing; including the importance of wearing the prescribed compression bandages, the need to elevate the legs when seated, the importance of exercise and so on. In the Mersey Region study most nurses had an understanding of the importance of lifestyle, diet and exercise, although the way in which this understanding was used to deliver advice to patients was not determined. Most community nurses (125; 86 per cent), (95 per cent confidence interval from 80 to 92 per cent), appreciated that leg elevation for patients with venous ulcers was important and said they gave this advice. More of the recently qualified nurses (n=77; 90 per cent) provided this information compared to community nurses who qualified before 1981 (n=47; 78 per cent). However some nurses did not realise that leg elevation was inadvisable for patients with arterial disease, as 45 (41 per cent of 111) nurses recommended that patients with arterial leg ulcers elevate their legs, inferring that this latter group did not fully appreciate the underlying pathology of the disease. This notion was further reinforced by the finding that only 53 (36 per cent) nurses recommended that patients with venous ulcers increase their level of exercise and mobility, suggesting that the majority may not fully understand the theory of the calf muscle pump (Roe et al, 1993).

Pain is an aspect of the care of patients with leg ulcers which often receives little attention. The Mersey Region survey asked community nurses about the advice given to patients regarding their pain; of the 66 nurses who reported they assessed patients' pain, only 42 per cent said they would follow it through with advice on analgesia (Roe et al, 1993). From the preliminary findings of a study that has investigated patients' perceptions of their leg ulcers, more than a third (n=33; 38 per cent) (sample = 88) of them found that pain was the worst thing they had to cope with, irrespective of the type of ulcer (see chapter 11). It would seem that the assessment of pain and subsequent advice about analgesia need greater emphasis in clinical practice.

PREVENTION AND REFERRAL

Few prospective studies have investigated the effectiveness of treatments in preventing re-ulceration; however, expert opinion deems that the wearing of compression hosiery after healing is an important means of reducing re-ulceration (see chapter 8). A 7 year follow-up of the 1981 Harrow prevalence survey was undertaken by Cornwall (1990). Of the original 123 patients, 109 agreed to be followed up and 119 limbs were found to have re-ulcerated. Cornwall suggests this was due to the fact that the compression hosiery available on prescription before 1988 was inadequate. It could have also been possible that even though compression hosiery had been prescribed for patients, it was not always worn. In the Mersey study the majority of nurses (n=92; 63 per cent) recognised the wearing of compression hosiery as an important preventative measure once the ulcer had healed, although it was unclear in this study that compression hosiery was being exclusively limited to patients with venous disease (Roe et al, 1993).

It is clear from a number of studies that the number of patients with leg ulceration who are referred for a specialist opinion appears low. The Northwick Park study (Cornwall et al, 1986) reported that 62 per cent of patients had never seen a specialist and 10 years later the Wirral study (Cullum and Last, 1993) found that only 41 per cent of patients had ever been referred to hospital. It is difficult to judge the appropriateness of these figures; there is no 'gold standard' referral rate and referral may be inappropriate or refused by the patient in a large number of cases. However, 77 patients in the Wirral study who had had a leg ulceration for 6 months or longer had never been referred. The importance of referring patients with non-healing or idiosyncratic ulceration needs to be emphasised to both nurses and general practitioners. Specialist assessment of a patient may isolate some hitherto unrecognised factor such as arterial insufficiency, or carcinoma (Ackroyd and Young, 1983). In the Mersey study 91 (63 per cent) (95 per cent confidence interval from 55 to 71 per cent) nurses would refer a patient whose ulcer was not healing for a medical opinion (Roe et al, 1993). As general practitioners tend to view the nurse as the leg ulcer expert and devolve treatment choice to her (Ertl, 1992), referral to the general practitioner may be insufficient and further referral to a consultant may also be necessary. In the Mersey study only one nurse mentioned referral as a measure to prevent re-ulceration (Roe et al, 1993).

CONSTRAINTS ON PRACTICE AND PROFESSIONAL ISSUES

It is appreciated that many factors influence nursing practice, not least the availability of resources. In the Mersey Region study community nurses were given an extensive list of possible constraints on their practice, and were asked to identify those which applied to them, and asked to note any others. The results are shown in table 10.4 (Roe and Luker, 1992). Most nurses were not constrained by nurse manager pressures or general practitioner pressures, although of the 11 (7 per cent) nurses who did feel constrained by their general practitioner, 10 of them qualified after 1981. Only a minority of nurses (n=31; 21 per cent) felt constrained by too few resources and this phenomenon was more commonly felt by nurses who had qualified post-1981 (n=24; 28 per cent) than before (n=6; 10 per cent). Similarly the majority of nurses (n=95; 66 per cent) were not constrained by difficulties in obtaining their preferred products; however fewer nurses who qualified before 1981 (n=13; 22 per cent), compared with those qualified post-1981 (n=37; 44 per cent) had such difficulties. Those more recently qualified were more likely to use 'modern' wound dressings and the problems may reflect the exclusion of products from the FP10 or, possibly, a general practitioner's reluctance to prescribe them. These factors would need further investigation. However, more than half of the nurses (n=81; 56 per cent) felt being able to *prescribe* wound care products would make a difference to the care they gave to their leg ulcer patients.

Table 10.4 Community nurse-identified constraints on practice

Identified constraints	Relevant sample
Caseload size	32
Under-staffing	67
Nurse manager pressures	10
Patient non-compliance	120
Patient's lifestyle	108
General practitioner pressures	11
Too few resources	31
Lack of supplies	30
Availability of preferred products	51
Lack of information	26
Lack of experience	18
Consultant's instructions	68
None of these	1
	n=146

The poor compliance of the leg ulcer patient is often blamed for poor healing rates (e.g. *Lancet*, 1982) and the nurse is able to promote compliance by educating and supporting the patient, and involving them in planning care (Poulton, 1991). In the Wirral study (Cullum and Last, 1993), each nurse was asked to rate the level of compliance of each individual leg ulcer patient in their care. Fifty six per cent of patients were regarded as very compliant, 33 per cent as of average compliance and only 11 per cent as poorly compliant. This contrasts with the findings of Roe and Luker (1992) who did not ask nurses about specific patients, but where 82 per cent of community nurses viewed poor patient compliance as a constraint to practice. The whole area of patient compliance and patient participation in leg ulcer care would benefit from more indepth study.

Continuing education and the proposed Post Registration Education and Practice Project (PREPP) (UKCC, 1989) will make it a professional requirement for all nurses to update their practice. Slightly more than half of the nurses (n=85; 58 per cent) in the Mersey Region study qualified after 1981 and had undertaken the more indepth syllabus for the district nurse qualification (Roe et al, 1993, 1994). It may be this factor which largely explains the significant differences found within the data on nurses' reported practice. Also, nurses who qualified more recently (n=59; 69 per cent) were more likely to have attended a course on leg ulcer management than those nurses who qualified before 1981 (n=5; 8 per cent). This finding was surprising, as one might expect that those nurses qualified the longest would be more likely to require and therefore attend an updating session. The more recently qualified nurses may have a greater appreciation of the need for continuing education, fostered by their initial preparation on the revised district nursing syllabus; however, it is impossible to say from this study. It is of some concern that community nurses who had been qualified the longest were least likely to have received any continuing education (Roe et al, 1993). None of the health authorities and trusts included in the Mersey Region study had a clinical nurse specialist for wound care or tissue viability. In recent years clinical nurse specialists for wound care and tissue viability have been appointed in an attempt to improve the dissemination of research and the quality of patient care (Cornwall et al, 1985).

Community nurses are generally more accessible to company representatives than hospital nurses. The majority of nurses (n=130; 89 per cent) in the Mersey Region study stated they used pharmaceutical company representatives as a source of information for their clinical practice (Roe et al, 1994). The influence of pharmaceutical company representatives has also been found in previous research, and manufacturer's recommendations and instructions often form the basis for nursing practice despite an absence of supporting research (Roe 1989). Luker and Kenrick (1992) have also found that drug representatives are viewed by community nurses as a source of scientific knowledge on which to base practice. Nurses should be dissuaded from relying on manufacturers as a predominant source of information and research findings as the information they provide is likely to be biased.

Nearly all of the nurses (n=134; 92 per cent) in the Mersey Region study stated that they had read journal articles about leg ulcer management within the previous year (Roe et al, 1994). However, even though professional and academic journals publish research findings, there is a wealth of published evidence, often conflicting results, and the primary research is often flawed in design. Anecdote is often presented as evidence for the effectiveness of a product, and it is difficult if not impossible for the practitioner to find a way through the quagmire of information with which they are presented. All health care should be based upon the most sound research evidence (Department of Health, 1991, 1992), and it is imperative that we look at ways of facilitating the development of research-based practice within nursing generally and for the management of patients with chronic leg ulcers in particular.

RECOMMENDATIONS FOR THE DEVELOPMENT OF PRACTICE

It is evident that all patients with chronic leg ulcers require an accurate medical diagnosis and comprehensive nursing assessment in order that the most appropriate care can be planned and delivered. It is essential that every patient's experience of pain is properly assessed and that patients are offered advice on analgesia and other methods of pain relief or else prescribed analgesia by the general practitioner. Appropriate advice about exercise and leg elevation should be given to patients with leg ulcers. Awareness amongst community nurses of the range of dressings and bandages available and their proper use must be increased.

It is recommended that members of the primary health care team and Information Pharmacists from Family Health Service Authorities develop practice guidelines for the management of patients with chronic leg ulcers. These guidelines should cover the assessment of patients and all aspects of treatment, and should include criteria to prompt the referral to specialists, of patients with non-healing ulcers or atypical clinical presentations. Such are the components of a high quality leg ulcer service.

Nursing has been slow to evaluate effective means of disseminating practice guidelines (incorporating research findings) to practitioners. Community nurses are particularly disadvantaged as they often work alone, with little or no access to library facilities and other educational resources. Educational initiatives such as study days, conferences, Clinical Information Packs (Kenrick et al, 1991), electronic publishing and television programmes such as the *Royal College of Nursing Nursing Update* series may be effective. It is important that senior management recognise the need of nursing, as well as medical personnel, to have time provided for study and updating. Expert clinicians such as Clinical Nurse Specialists in Tissue Viability or Leg Ulcer Care are in a position to act as resources, and to provide the essential teaching of basic clinical skills, such as the application of compression bandaging, and patient assessment, in the clinical area.

SUMMARY

This chapter has reviewed a number of key studies which have investigated the nursing management of leg ulcers. A number of recommendations for the development of nursing practice have been made and include:

●   Patients should receive an initial medical examination and diagnosis as well as a comprehensive nursing assessment.
●   An objective assessment of pain should be part of the nursing assessment—

appropriate advice regarding analgesia or referral to the general practitioner should be given if pain is a feature.

● Research-based clinical guidelines for the management of patients with leg ulcers should be compiled by primary health care teams.

● Nurses also require clinically-based education regarding assessment and management, including the correct application of compression bandaging and use of doppler ultrasound.

● Criteria for the referral of patients should be part of these clinical guidelines.

It is essential that basic nurse education programmes, which now prepare nurses for practice in the community, cover the management of leg ulcers, and the theory and practice of bandaging. Other key educational developments would include the evaluation of methods of research dissemination and the application of those found to be effective, and the statutory provision of time for nurses to update their knowledge.

References

Ackroyd J S, Young A E (1983) Leg Ulcers that do not heal. *British Medical Journal*, **286**: 207–208.

Blair S D, Wright D D, Backhouse C M, Riddle E and McCollum C N (1988) Sustained compression and the healing of chronic venous ulcers. *British Medical Journal*, **297**: 1159–1161.

British Medical Journal (1977) Topical antibiotics. *British Medical Journal*, **1**: 1494.

Browse N L, Burnand K G and Lea Thomas M (1988) *Diseases of the Veins: Pathology, Diagnosis and Treatment*. London: Edward Arnold.

Callam M J, Ruckley C V, Harper D R and Dale J J (1985) Chronic ulceration of the leg: extent of the problem and provision of care. *British Medical Journal*, **290**: 1855–1856.

Cameron J (1990) Patch testing for leg ulcer patients. *Nursing Times*, **85**(25): 63–64.

Cornwall J V (1985) Leg Ulcer Specialist. *Journal of District Nursing*, **4**(3): 4–11.

Cornwall J (1990) Update on leg ulcer survey. *Journal of District Nursing*, **8**(11): 9–10.

Cornwall J V, Dore C J and Lewis J D (1986) Leg ulcers: epidemiology and aetiology. *British Journal of Surgery*, **73**: 693–696.

Cullum N A and Last S (1993) The prevalence, characteristics and management of leg ulcers in a UK community. *2nd European Conference on Advances in Wound Management*, Harrogate.

Cullum N (1994) *The Nursing Management of Leg Ulcers in the Community: A Critical Review of Research*. Department of Nursing, University of Liverpool, report submitted to the Department of Health.

Department of Health (1991) *Research for Health*. London: Department of Health Research and Development Division.

Department of Health (1992) *Assessing the Effects of Health Technologies*. London: Department of Health.

Ertl (1992) A recipe for assessment. *Journal of District Nursing*, July: 10–14.

Gibson B (1990) Use of compression in the treatment of leg ulcers. *Care, Science and Practice*, **8**(2): 67–69.

Gilchrist B (1989) The treatment of leg ulcers with occlusive hydrocolloid dressings: a microbiological study. In: *Directions in Nursing Research*, eds Wilson Barnett J and Robinson S, pp. 51–58. London: Scutari.

Journal of District Nursing (1986) Your data on leg ulcers. *Journal District Nursing*, **5**(9): 53–56.

Kenrick M, Luker K, Cullum N and Roe B (1991) *Clinical Information Pack No. 1—The Management of Leg Ulcers in the Community*. Liverpool: Department of Nursing, University of Liverpool.

Lancet (1982) Diagnosis and treatment of venous ulceration. *Lancet*, **ii**: 247–248.

Leaper D (1986) Antiseptics and their effect on healing tissue. *Nursing Times*, **82**(22): 45–47.

Luker K A and Kenrick M (1992) An exploratory study of the sources of influence on the clinical decisions of community nurses. *Journal of Advanced Nursing*, **17**: 457–466.

Mallett J and Charles H (1990) Defining the leg ulcer problem. *Journal District Nursing*, **July**: 5–10.

Panel of Assessors for District Nurse Training (1976) *Report on the Education and Training of District Nurses*. London: Department of Health.

Poulton B (1991) Factors which influence patient compliance. *Journal of Tissue Viability*, **1**: 108–110.

Roe B H (1989) Use of bladder washouts: a study of nurses' recommendations. *Journal of Advanced Nursing*, **14**: 494–500.

Roe B H and Luker K A (1992) *Study of the Nursing Management of Patients with Leg Ulcers in the Community*. Report to Mersey Regional Health Authority. Department of Nursing, University of Liverpool.

Roe B H, Luker K A, Cullum N A, Griffiths J M and Kenrick M (1993) Assessment, prevention and monitoring of chronic leg ulcers in the community: report of a survey. *Journal of Clinical Nursing*, **2**(5): 299–306.

Roe B H, Griffiths J M, Kenrick M, Cullum N A and Hutton J (1994) Nursing treatment of patients with chronic leg ulcers in the community: report of a survey. *Journal of Clinical Nursing* **3**(3) 159–168.

Sleigh J W and Winter S P K (1985) Hazards of hydrogen peroxide. *British Medical Journal*, **291**: 6510, 1706.

Thomas S (1990) *Wound Management and Dressings*. London: The Pharmaceutical Press.

UKCC (1989) *Post Registration Education and Practice Project*. London: UKCC.

11

Patients' Perceptions of

Chronic Leg Ulceration

INTRODUCTION

Recent changes in the Health Service and the development of *The Patient's Charter* (Department of Health, 1991) have placed increased emphasis on identifying the health needs of patients and consumers' views in relation not only to the service, but also to the care they receive. These timely developments intend that patients and clients participate in their care and that their views are heard. Patients are encouraged to be active participants in their care, rather than passive recipients. Most research in the management of patients with leg ulcers has examined the effectiveness of treatments; however, the human costs for the individual with a leg ulcer in relation to pain, decreased mobility and social isolation have not been fully investigated.

This chapter presents a review of key research into patients' perceptions of chronic leg ulcers and its impact on well-being and lifestyle. Recommendations for the future development of clinical practice are also presented.

REVIEW OF KEY RESEARCH

Context

It is commonly believed that many patients with leg ulcers do not want their ulcer to heal, as they would lose the social contact with community nurses and visits to the leg ulcer clinic (Muir Gray, 1983, Ryan, 1987, Browse et al, 1988). It has been reported, largely on the basis of anecdote, that some patients tamper with their bandages and dressings in order to prevent healing; a phenomenon termed 'the knitting needle syndrome' (Moffatt et al, 1991). In a study to evaluate the effectiveness of community leg ulcer clinics, Moffatt et al (1991) found that patients with leg ulcers not only experienced pain and worry as a consequence of having a leg ulcer, but that it also interfered with their ability to perform housework and engage in a social life. The Symptom Rating Test, a validated measure of psychiatric morbidity (Kellner, 1986) was used by Moffatt et al (1991) to measure anxiety, depression, hostility and cognition. They found that anxiety, depression, hostility and cognition all improved over the 12 weeks that patients attended the new community leg ulcer clinics, and that a significant decrease in levels of depression occurred in patients whose ulcers healed. As this was an uncontrolled study these positive effects cannot be confidently attributed to the new intervention, and could have been due to a Hawthorn effect. In the Lothian and Forth Valley Project, Callam et al (1988) interviewed and examined 600 patients with chronic leg ulcers. They found that having a leg ulcer either moderately or severely affected the work and leisure activities of 42 per cent of patients, with a further 10 per cent reporting that it impaired their mobility. However, levels of mobility and measures of health for leg ulcer patients have not been compared to those of age-matched individuals without leg ulcers. Social isolation and loneliness have also been suggested as explanations for patients not complying with leg ulcer treatments (Muir Gray and Wilcock, 1981; Smith, 1982; Millard, 1984; Moody, 1984; Wise, 1986a, b). However, these remain theories yet to be proven. An exploration of the psychological and social impact of having a leg ulcer is very much needed.

Current Research

A study was undertaken by the authors to investigate patients' perceptions of their leg ulcers and the impact of having a leg ulcer on their well-being and lifestyle. A random sample of 88 patients aged 65 and over with leg ulcers was recruited from the community of Wirral Health Authority. A semi-structured interview was undertaken with these patients, and a variety of data collected including demographic, functional (e.g. level of mobility) and experiential. Patients' feelings and knowledge about their ulcer were also explored. Established health measures were also used including the Nottingham Health Profile (Hunt et al, 1981), The Life Satisfaction Index (Morgan et al, 1987), The Hospital Anxiety and Depression Scale (Zigmond and Snaithe, 1983), and the short form McGill Pain Questionnaire (Melzack, 1987). The Health Locus of Control (Wallston et al, 1976a, b) was also used to determine how patients perceive and cope with their illness. People who expect that their own behaviour influences health outcomes are said to have an 'internal locus of control', whilst those who believe outside forces have a greater influence have 'external control' (Rotter, 1966). Orientation in health locus of control has been linked with levels of compliance (Shillinger, 1983; Balsmeyer, 1984; Hussey and Gilliland, 1989). Each leg ulcer was traced and photographed against a measuring scale. The ankle:brachial pressure index (ABPI) was recorded using a Mini Doppler (Huntleigh Technology Ltd) and sphygmomanometer.

The measures of health and quality of life, described above, were compared with those in a population of similar age without leg ulcers, obtained from the well-elderly population via the Family Health Services Authority (FHSA) and practice nurses. Seven practice nurses agreed to include the measures of health and quality of life as part of their over-75s health screening ($n = 70$). All data collected were coded and entered into SPSS/PC for analysis. A selection of the results are presented.

BIOGRAPHICAL DETAILS

A total of 88 patients with chronic leg ulcers (mean age 80 years, range 65–98) and 60 control subjects without leg ulcers (mean age 77 years, range 65–91) participated. Age and sex were similarly represented in each group (table 11.1). The majority of leg ulcer patients (n = 64; 73 per cent) were widowed and 53 per cent (n = 47) lived alone. Seventy three per cent (n = 64) of patients had leg ulcers on their left leg, 58 per cent (n = 51) on their right leg and 15 per cent (n = 13) of patients had ulcers on both legs. According to the researcher (CH), 24 per cent (n = 21) of patients had ulcers that smelt unpleasant.

Table 11.1 Age and sex characteristics of leg ulcer patients and control group

	Leg ulcer patients (n = 88)	Control group (n = 60)
Mean age (years)	80	77
Standard deviation	6.58	6.72
Range	65–98	65–91
Sex: male	30 (34%)	24 (40%)
Sex: female	58 (66%)	36 (60%)

Knowledge of Leg Ulcers

The majority of patients (n = 73; 84 per cent) were able to locate their leg ulcers whilst the remainder could not due to poor eyesight, lack of knowledge, lack of interest or denial. Patients had their ulcers for between 3 months and 4 years (table 11.2), with 59 per cent (n = 51) of patients reporting that this ulcer was the first they had ever experienced. When asked for the cause of the ulcer, 55 per cent (n = 48) of patients felt their ulcer was the result of trauma, 21 per cent (n = 18) due to an underlying medical condition, whilst 20 per cent (n = 17) did not know or could not remember the cause of their ulcer. The majority of patients (n = 53; 60 per cent) said they would not like any more information about their ulcer. This is contrary to other client groups with a chronic condition, such as patients using long-term indwelling urethral catheterisation (Roe and Brocklehurst, 1987), and could have important implications for the design of materials for patient education. Of those who would have liked more information (n = 34, 40 per cent),

Table 11.2 Duration of this episode of ulceration

Time	No. of patients
3–6 months	12 (14%)
7–12 months	13 (15%)
1–2 years	17 (20%)
2–4 years	20 (23%)
> 4 years	25 (29%)
Total	87

the type of information required related to the cause of the ulcer, care of the ulcer, how long the ulcer would last and how the ulcer would affect their lives.

PATIENT'S FEELINGS

The leg ulcer was a source of worry to the majority of patients (n = 79; 90 per cent). Pain (n = 33; 38 per cent), restricted mobility (n = 27; 31 per cent), the inconvenience of dressings (n = 9), exudate (n = 7), and worry about healing (n = 3) were variously described as the worst thing about having an ulcer. The majority of patients (n = 62; 71 per cent) expressed negative feelings about having an ulcer:

"It makes me into an invalid."
"I hate knowing there is something wrong with me."

However, eight patients said their ulcer did not bother them and for four patients it was not their worst problem. Some people were just resigned to having an ulcer (n = 13; 15 per cent), whilst 10 patients said there *were* good things about having an ulcer:

"I get meals on wheels now."
"I like to see the District Nurses."

This last comment supports the notion of patients benefiting from the social contact of the district nurses.

All but one patient was aware of their ulcer; 42 per cent (n = 36) all of the time, 24 per cent (n = 21) most of the time and 35 per cent (n = 30) occasionally. Twenty nine per cent (n = 25) of patients were most aware of their ulcer at night. Forty nine per cent (n = 43) of patients felt that other people noticed their ulcer, which was upsetting for some patients (n = 24; 55 per cent) but of no bother to others (n = 19; 56 per cent). Patients who felt that other people noticed their leg ulcer had significantly lower Life Satisfaction scores (ANOVA, $P < 0.05$). However, 77 per cent (n = 67) of patients did feel that their ulcer was getting better.

LIFESTYLE

Most patients with leg ulcers were able to walk with or without the use of aids and appliances (n = 66; 76 per cent) or with the help of another person (n = 13; 15 per cent). Eighty two per cent (n = 71) of patients had full use of both hands and 75 per cent (n = 65) were able to see using spectacles. The majority of patients (n = 86; 99 per cent) had retired from employment, with seven patients having retired due to the ill health caused by their ulcer. These seven patients retired when their mobility had deteriorated to the extent that they were no longer able to perform in jobs such as those of security guard, road sweeper and dance teacher.

The typical patient was in contact with relatives and friends on a daily basis, district nurses two to three times a week and their general practitioner less than once a month (table 11.3).

Table 11.3 Amount and type of social contact for patients with leg ulceration

Type	daily	two to three times per week	weekly	monthly	less than monthly	never
Friends	21	20	26	8	5	7
Relatives	31	15	16	8	0	17
District nurse	9	53	18	1	0	6
General practitioner	0	0	0	9	65	13
Home help	5	21	8	0	0	53
Other community services	2	3	1	0	0	81
Other	0	3	1	0	0	83

Total = 87.

Sixty two per cent (n = 71) of patients went out of their home on a daily basis or a number of times per week and were therefore considered able to get about. On these outings patients visited friends or relatives (n = 44; 51 per cent), shops (n = 35; 41 per cent), their general practitioner (n = 26; 30 per cent), the day centre (n = 8), a variety of different places, such as the church, the pub or went out purely for exercise (n = 22; 25 per cent). However, the majority of them (n = 70; 80 per cent) felt they were going out less frequently as a result of their ulcer, due to the pain and discomfort experienced (n = 39; 56 per cent), reduced mobility (n = 13; 15 per cent), time spent waiting for the district nurse to call (n = 6; 7 per cent) or as a result of embarrassment (n = 4; 5 per cent).

Some patients felt that having a leg ulcer had affected their contact with friends (n = 24; 27 per cent) and family (n = 18; 20 per cent) due to a decrease in their mobility. Seventy per cent (n = 60) of people with leg ulcers had been able to maintain their hobbies, although 43 per cent (n = 37) had given some of them up as a result of their leg ulcer causing decreased mobility or increased pain, which affected their concentration. Typical comments given included;

"I can't get my waders on to go fishing."
"I can't get my legs wet in the swimming baths."

In relation to washing and dressing, 90 per cent (n = 78) of patients said that having a leg ulcer caused them problems with washing and bathing, usually because they could not get their leg ulcer wet (n = 62; 78 per cent). Leg ulcers caused problems with dressing in 82 per cent (n = 71) of patients; due to ill-fitting footwear (n = 55; 78 per cent) or problems getting clothes on and off (n = 16; 18 per cent). Some patients found difficulty in performing other activities of daily living such as preparing meals or carrying out housework, due to the decreased mobility caused by their leg ulcer (n = 65 [75 per cent] for preparing a meal and n = 75 [87 per cent] for housework).

Eighteen per cent (n = 16) of patients with leg ulcers were also carers and having a leg ulcer had affected the ability of 10 of them to perform as carers. This was significantly associated with a raised level of anxiety (ANOVA, $P<0.05$). All of these people expressed negative feelings about their impaired ability to be a carer;

"I feel guilty as I can't walk the dog."
"I'm embarrassed that my husband has to do everything."

Seventy four per cent ($n = 65$) of patients with leg ulcers found that it affected their sleep, which for the majority ($n = 61$, 69 per cent) was due to the pain and discomfort. Herr (1992) also found disturbed sleep in the elderly is commonly associated with leg pain. In our present study a minority of patients with leg ulcers ($n = 3$) also felt that their sex life had been impaired as a consequence of their leg ulcer. It is apparent therefore that having a leg ulcer may have a very limiting effect on one's lifestyle, one's ability to undertake routine activities of daily living and to be a carer.

HEALTH MEASURES

The health locus of control was used to determine the health orientation of patients with leg ulcers, and their scores were compared with those from other populations. The mean locus of control score for the patients with leg ulcers in this study was 45.7 (standard deviation [SD] 8.7). Leg ulcer patients were more externally orientated compared with the community residents (mean 35.9, SD 7.1) and hypertensive outpatients (mean 40.1, SD 6.2) quoted in the literature (Wallston et al, 1976a, b). This indicates that, in general, patients with leg ulcers have a generalised expectancy that those factors which control their health are ones over which they have little control.

The Nottingham Health Profile was used to measure perceived pain, loss of energy, emotional reactions, problems with sleep, physical mobility and social isolation for both leg ulcer patients and the control group. The mean score for the amount of perceived pain experienced by leg ulcer patients was 45.06 (SD 32.47) and for the controls was 15.51 (SD 21.44). Patients with leg ulcers had significantly higher scores for perceived pain than the controls (by independent t-test, $P<0.05$; 95 per cent confidence interval from 20.73 to 38.37 per cent). The intensity of pain at the time of the interview increased according to the size of the ulcer by simple linear regression ($P=0.04$), indicating that larger ulcers were more painful than smaller ulcers.

Pain was also examined using the shortened form of the McGill Pain Questionnaire, which measures the type and intensity of pain. The majority of leg ulcer patients ($n = 61$; 70 per cent) described their pain as 'aching', whilst the highest mean intensity (2.16) related to a feeling of 'sharp' pain (table 11.4). At the time of the interview, 31 per cent ($n = 27$) of patients were experiencing pain from their leg ulcer; 11 per cent ($n = 9$) of patients had mild pain, 13 per cent ($n = 11$) discomforting pain and 8 per cent ($n = 7$) had distressing pain. The intensity of pain was inversely proportional to the ABPI, supporting the notion that ulcers with an arterial component are more painful (ANOVA, $P < 0.05$).

The amount of energy loss experienced by leg ulcer patients, as measured by the Nottingham Health Profile (mean 58.30, SD 38.85) was significantly greater than for the control group (mean 24.26, SD 26.34) (independent t-test, $P<0.05$; 95

Table 11.4   Pain reported using the McGill Pain Questionnaire

Pain description	No. of patients (%)	Mean intensity
Throbbing	48 (55)	1.89
Shooting	34 (39)	1.85
Stabbing	26 (30)	1.97
Sharp	24 (28)	2.16
Cramping	11 (13)	1.92
Gnawing	10 (11)	2.10
Hot-burning	37 (43)	2.03
Aching	61 (70)	2.05
Heavy	37 (43)	1.63
Tender	38 (44)	1.98
Splitting	9 (19)	1.80
Tiring	41 (47)	1.95
Sickening	15 (17)	1.87
Fearful	2 (2)	1.00
Punishing	4 (5)	2.00
	$n = 88$	

per cent confidence interval from 23.26 to 44.82 per cent). No difference was found in the mean scores for perceived emotional reaction to health between the leg ulcer patients (mean 22.99, SD 28.36) and the control group (mean 17.47, SD 21.42).

More patients with leg ulcers identified health factors as causing problems with looking after their home, their social life, home life and hobbies and interests than the control group (independent t-test, $P<0.05$) (table 11.5). Patients with leg ulcers also had significantly lower scores for life satisfaction (mean 14.87, SD 4.95) than the control group (mean 16.98, SD 4.78) (independent t-test, $P<0.05$; 95 per cent confidence interval from 0.35 to 3.87 per cent). Using the Hospital Anxiety and Depression scale no difference in anxiety was found between patients with leg ulcers and the control group. However, there were more depressed patients with leg ulcers than without (independent t-test, $P<0.01$; 95 per cent confidence interval for this difference is from 0.3 to 2.2 per cent). Patients with malodorous ulcers had higher anxiety and depression scores, lower life satisfaction and less social contact (independent t-test, $P<0.05$). A significant relationship was also found between patients going out of their house less frequently because of their leg ulcer, and high anxiety scores and lower life satisfaction (ANOVA, $P<0.05$).

Table 11.5   Problems experienced by leg ulcer patients and people without leg ulcers (Nottingham Health Profile)

Problems with	Leg ulcer patients (%)	Control group (%)
Work	15 (17)	5 (8)
Looking after the home	55 (63)	18 (30)*
Social life	55 (63)	16 (27)
Home life	35 (40)	6 (10)*
Sex life	9 (10)	6 (10)
Interests and hobbies	43 (49)	16 (27)*
Holidays	34 (39)	17 (28)
	$n = 87$	$n = 60$

* $P < 0.01$.

MANAGEMENT OF THE ULCER

The majority of patients (n = 81; 92 per cent) had their leg ulcers dressed in their own home, predominantly by the district nurse (n = 79; 90 per cent). Only one patient felt that this was inconvenient because they had to wait in all day and would have preferred to attend a clinic for their dressing. Fifty eight per cent (n = 51) of patients receiving district nursing visits were mobile with or without aids, and perhaps could have attended a local clinic or general practitioner's surgery. The majority of patients found their dressings (n = 70; 81 per cent) and bandages (n = 63; 78 per cent) comfortable; however, it is of note that only four patients were receiving compression bandages. Twenty three per cent (n = 20) of patients said they sometimes removed 'uncomfortable' stockings and bandages, because they were too loose, too tight or too hot. On the whole, most patients (n = 81; 92 per cent) where satisfied with their treatment. However patients' expectations of healing were not investigated, and it is not known if the relatively high level of satisfaction was based on low expectations.

RECOMMENDATIONS FOR THE DEVELOPMENT OF PRACTICE

Most people with leg ulcers are elderly and approximately half in this study lived alone. A large proportion (20 per cent) of patients did not know what had caused their ulcer, having an ulcer was a source of worry for most people and yet the majority (60 per cent) said that they did not want more information about the ulcer. This is surprising and perhaps depends on an individual's interpretation of the word 'information' within the context of the interview. We would suggest that the need for more 'therapeutic' communication between leg ulcer patients and the primary health care team has been highlighted. It is also important to remember that individuals will have varying requirements for both the depth and the packaging of the information.

The impact of pain on individuals with leg ulcers has emerged strongly from many aspects of this study, and has previously been underestimated. The management of patients' pain must be improved, as discussed in chapter 10.

Few patients (n = 10) reported that having a leg ulcer conferred any benefits whatsoever. Those benefits reported included the provision of Meals on Wheels and the visits of the district nurse; however, it could be argued that individuals with a propensity to look on the bright side would be likely to perceive benefits. Conversely others may not be willing to disclose perceived benefits to a stranger within the context of a fairly structured interview. Further study using a qualitative methodology would be required to gain further understanding of many of these issues.

The patients in this study were surprisingly mobile, as 76 per cent were described as mobile with or without aids; however, most reported that they went out less frequently as a result of the ulcer. The Riverside model of community leg ulcer clinics (chapter 12) would provide the opportunity for both exercise and social interaction, as well as saving money in district nurse travelling time.

The fact that most patients were satisfied with care and found their bandages comfortable may be due to their poor expectations of healing, and the lack of provision of compression bandages. These two issues are intimately connected. Patients in this study, randomly selected from the population of elderly people with leg ulcers, had ulcers of duration 3 months to 4 years. It has been shown by Moffatt et al (1991) and others that over 60 per cent of leg ulcers in people of this age group can be completely healed within 12 weeks using compression bandaging. However, only seven individuals in this study were receiving any form of compression. Most patients wore a straight tubular bandage (32 per cent), elastocrepe alone (20 per cent) or a crepe bandage (15 per cent). Fifteen individuals wore no bandage or stocking, thus a large proportion of patients, most of whom would have venous ulcers, did not receive a bandage or stocking capable of delivering sustained graduated compression. One is driven to suggest that if patients were thoroughly and accurately assessed, and given the appropriate treatment, most ulcers would heal fairly quickly and many of those factors which diminish their quality of life would disappear with the ulcer.

SUMMARY

This chapter has reviewed the literature in relation to patients' experience of their leg ulcer, and has presented a study which investigated patients' perceptions of their leg ulcer and its impact on their well-being and lifestyle. A number of recommendations for the development of clinical practice have been made, including the importance of recognising the impact of a leg ulcer on the individual, the effects leg ulceration has on patients' lives and the importance of recognising the potential need for pain control and assistance with activities of daily living. The amount of worry that leg ulceration causes for patients should be recognised, and strategies developed to diminish this. The organisation of care should be reviewed, and the most cost-effective system, which meets both the needs of the health service and the patient should be selected (see chapter 12). Strategies should be developed to enable patients to actively participate in their care.

References

Balsmeyer B (1984) Locus of control and the use of strategies to promote self care. *Journal of Community Health Nursing*, **3**: 171–179.
Browse N L, Burnand K G and Lea Thomas M (1988) *Diseases of the Veins: Pathology, Diagnosis and Treatment*. London: Edward Arnold.
Callam M J, Harper D R, Dale J J and Ruckley C V (1988) Chronic leg ulceration: socio-economic aspects. *Scottish Medical Journal*, **33**: 358–360.
Department of Health (1991) *The Patients' Charter*. London: HMSO.
Herr K A (1992) Night leg pain in the elderly. *Geriatric Nursing*, **13**(1): 13–16.
Hunt S M, McKenna S P, McEwan J, Williams J and Papp E (1981) The Nottingham Health

Profile: subjective health status and medical consultations. *Social Science and Medicine*, **15a**: 221–229.

Hussey L C and Gilliland K (1989) Compliance, low literacy and locus of control. *Nursing Clinics of North America*, **24**: 605–611.

Kellner R (1986) The symptom rating test. In: *Assessment of Depression*, eds Sartorius N and Ban T. New York: Springer.

Melzack R (1987) The short-form McGill pain questionnaire: major properties and scoring methods. *Pain*, **1**: 277–299.

Millard L (1984) Dermatological pathomimicry. *Lancet*, **ii**: 970.

Moffatt C J, Franks P J, Bosanquet N, Oldroyd M, Connolly M, Brown P, O'Malley M K, Greenhalgh R and McCollum C N (1991) *The Provision of Innovation in Venous Ulcer Management to the Elderly Population in the Community*. Report to the King Edward's Hospital Fund for London.

Moody M (1984) A new lease of life. *Nursing Times*, **July 4**: 46.

Morgan K, Dallasso H M, Arie T, Byrne E J, Jones R and Waite J (1987) Mental health and psychological well-being among the old and the very old living at home. *British Journal of Psychiatry*, **150**: 801–807.

Muir Gray J A (1983) Social aspects of peripheral vascular disease. In: *Peripheral Vascular Disease in the Elderly*, ed. McCarthy S T, pp. 191–199. London: Churchill Livingstone.

Muir Gray J A and Wilcock G (1981) *Our elders*. Oxford: Oxford University Press.

Roe B H and Brocklehurst J C (1987) The study of patients with long term indwelling urethral catheters. *Journal of Advanced Nursing*, **19**: 713–714.

Rotter J B (1966) Generalised expectancies for internal versus external control of reinforcement. *Psychology Monographs: General and Applied*, **80**: 100–127.

Ryan T J (1987) *The Management of Leg Ulcers*, 2nd edn. Oxford: Oxford Medical Publications.

Shillinger F L (1983) Locus of control implications for nursing practice. *Journal of Nursing Scholarship*, **15**(2): 58–63.

Smith M (1982) Nursing management of the leg ulcer in the community. *Nursing Times*, **July 21**: 1228–1232.

Wallston K A, Kaplan G D and Maides S A (1976a) Development and validation of the Health Locus of Control Scale. *Journal of Consulting and Clinical Psychology*, **44**: 580–585.

Wallston K A, Maides S A and Wallston B S (1976b) Health-related information seeking as a function of health-related locus of control and health value. *Journal of Research in Personality*, **10**: 215–222.

Wise G (1986a) The social ulcer. *Nursing Times*, **May 21**: 47–49.

Wise G (1986b) Overcoming loneliness. *Nursing Times*, **May 28**: 37–42.

Zigmond A S and Snaith R P (1983) The hospital anxiety and depression scale. *Acta Psychiatrica Scandinavica*, **150**: 801–807.

12

The Organisation and

Delivery of Leg Ulcer Care

INTRODUCTION

Recent epidemiological studies suggest that between 75 000 and 90 000 patients are receiving treatment for a chronic venous ulcer at any one time (Callam et al, 1985, Cornwall et al, 1986). However, these studies may have underestimated the problem as they only identified patients attending a health professional for treatment. Recent work within Riverside Health Authority identified a further 25 per cent of patients not receiving medical or nursing care prior to attending a community leg ulcer clinic (Moffatt et al, 1992). This clearly represents an unmet need in the community.

No studies have been published to determine the precise incidence of new ulceration, although information is available on the incidence of re-ulceration. The Forth and Lothian Study identified that two-thirds of patients had already had more than one episode of ulceration at the time of their assessment (Callam et al, 1985). Of the remainder approximately 50 per cent had had their ulcer for more than 1 year. A similar figure was identified within the Harrow Study (Cornwall et al, 1986).

In a hospital dermatology clinic, 69 patients with recently healed ulcers were fitted with compression stockings. Of the total, 69 per cent of limbs re-ulcerated within 1 year of healing (Monk and Sarkay, 1982). In a randomized controlled trial of oxerutins versus placebo, in 138 patients with newly healed ulcers, no overall difference was found in the recurrence rate between the groups, but the re-ulceration rate in the placebo group was 22 per cent at 1 year, rising to 32 per cent at 18 months (Wright et al, 1991). Both these studies indicate that even when an ulcer heals, there is a high risk of re-ulceration. The treatment of leg ulceration is essentially a community problem, and patients are managed by the primary care team and in particular the district or practice nurses.

Less than 1 per cent of leg ulcer patients are treated on an inpatient basis, although when this does occur it is often for extended periods and the cost per patient is high (Callam et al, 1985). A recent study indicated £89 million was spent in 1989 on inpatient care alone (Laing, 1992). The Harrow Study identified 62 per cent of patients who had never been referred for a specialist opinion despite the longevity of ulceration (Cornwall et al, 1986). Those patients who attend hospital outpatients are seen by a variety of specialists and often require much additional support from the community nursing service (Callam et al, 1985).

A recent survey of district nurses indicated that 98 per cent had responsibility for leg ulcer patients (*Journal of District Nursing*, 1987) and that many decisions in treatment were delegated to the nurse (McIntosh, 1979). Evidence suggests that district nurses spend between 25 and 50 per cent of their time caring for these patients (Moffatt et al, 1992), half of whom are seen more than twice weekly and one-fifth daily (Callam et al, 1985). Despite these facts, there is a distinct lack of training in leg ulcer management either pre- or post-registration.

Until recently, few attempts have been made to estimate the problem of leg ulceration in terms of community and acute resources. Information gained from the Riverside study estimated the cost of treating leg ulcers within the district prior to establishing community ulcer clinics to be £400 000 for a population of 250 000 (Bosanquet, 1992). This extrapolates to a minimum of £400 million spent annually on leg ulceration in the UK, with little evidence that the situation is improving. The increasing number of elderly people in society is likely to lead to a growing demand for treatment, a corresponding increase in cost and an elderly population who may be less tolerant of chronic disabling conditions such as leg ulceration.

TACKLING THE PROBLEM

The treatment of leg ulcers is considered to provide few benefits for patients or staff (Bosanquet, 1992). Many community patients are frail and immobile, with a multiplicity of problems and remain on the district nursing register for many years (Antrobus, 1987). These factors can lead to low staff morale and poor motivation when faced with patients with long-standing, non-healing ulcers. This may also be true for the patients, who become disillusioned and non-compliant when treatment regimes are unsuccessful. This leads to a high level of dependency on the community services, which a patient may find difficult to relinquish when the ulcer heals. The ulcer *may* then be viewed as an asset (Wise, 1986) (see chapter 11).

One problem facing those involved in the management of leg ulcers has been the lack of objective means of determining the likely cause of ulceration (Cornwall et al, 1986). Doppler ultrasound is a very useful tool for detecting arterial disease but it is still not widely available in the community and assessment of the patient's arterial status is often made by observation alone. Recent studies have identified that at least 10 per cent of patients with leg ulceration have an impaired arterial circulation, and this may occur concurrently with venous disease and other pathologies (Cornwall et al, 1986). In a study within Riverside Health Authority, 37 per cent of all patients would have received incorrect treatment if Doppler ultrasound had not been available to check the patient's arterial status.

Of the many hundreds of products used on leg ulcers, many are totally inappropriate (Vydelingum, 1990) and few treatment regimes are based on sound scientific research. There is evidence that aggressive advertising changes the pattern of use of dressings, irrespective of efficacy (Bale, 1989). The Harrow Study identified 90 agents in use in 108 different ways on the ulcer or surrounding skin (Cornwall et al, 1986). Many topical agents are detrimental, and lead to contact dermatitis. Ryan reports that 80 per cent of patients with a leg ulcer for more than 5 years are sensitive to at least one topical agent used in ulcer care (Ryan, 1983).

In recent years graduated compression has come to be recognised as the most important conservative treatment of venous ulcers (Sigg, 1963; Meyerovitz and Nelson, 1964; Sigel et al, 1973; Blair et al, 1988). Bandages available in the community on prescription have been incapable of applying sustained compression due to their inelasticity and this is a major reason why venous ulcers remain an intractable problem (Thomas, 1990). The last decade has seen the development of elastic bandages containing synthetic elastomeric fibres, which can maintain a defined level of compression (Moffatt, 1992). Changes in the drug tariff should allow these to be widely available in the community. This will however increase the risk of inappropriate use of compression in patients with arterial disease. One study identified 147 cases of compression damage during a 5 year period. Of these seven required arterial reconstruction and 12 amputation (Callam et al, 1987).

Although the provision of leg ulcer care in this country has been described as uncoordinated and generally ineffective (Cornwall et al, 1986; Bosanquet, 1992), centres of excellence do exist in the UK in both the acute and community services. However, these are isolated, with the majority of health authorities lacking strategies for the management of these patients. Initiatives in leg ulcer management have tended to spring from hospital specialist centres where liaison with the surrounding community has been developed.

Lewis and Cornwall (1987) demonstrated that effective assessment and treatment resulted in improved ulcer healing. The Harrow Study offered support and referral of patients from the community to a vascular unit, as well as domiciliary visitation. A long established programme exists in Lothian and Forth Valley, with an international reputation for excellence in clinical research in venous disease. Oxford have demonstrated the effective use of dermatology support in providing a comprehensive service to the community, including a patch testing service for patients (Cameron, 1990).

Community leg ulcer clinics have been established in a number of areas in this country (Hedges and Stubbings, 1991; Eagle, 1992; Russell and Bowles 1992, Griffey 1992). They have been shown to use community nurse time effectively. Improved healing is largely dependent on the use of effective research-based treatment regimes.

The formation of resource groups and standardisation of protocols by Ertl has resulted in effective district nurse management of patients in Eastbourne (Ertl, 1992). Similar initiatives in Parkside have demonstrated improved ulcer healing rates when a short-stretch compression regime was implemented in a small study in the community (Charles, 1991).

The role of the wound care specialist continues to evolve. A growing number of districts are employing nurses to develop wound care as a speciality. These nurses have responsibility for facilitating research-based practice and providing educational support to all nurses working in the clinical areas; however, little education or support exists to prepare nurse specialists for this demanding role.

The role of general practitioners in leg ulcer care has remained small, with most relying on the skills of practice nurses or district nurses (Robinson, 1990). Wound care is inadequately taught at medical schools, leaving doctors ill-prepared to deal with these patients (Bennett, 1992).

Anomalies still exist between hospital and community (Cockbill, 1992). Many of the dressings used in hospitals are not available within the community, which leads to frustration and poor continuity of treatment. Community restraints may make treatments requested by hospitals inappropriate for community nurses to use.

Whilst the provision of effective care remains patchy in this country, there is a growing awareness of the enormity of the problem and the financial implications. The demand for educational programmes to equip nurses with the skills and knowledge to implement research-based practice far outstrips the resources available. There is no national co-ordination in this area and the impact of individual centres will remain small unless such a strategy is adopted.

THE RIVERSIDE COMMUNITY LEG ULCER PROJECT

Research conducted by the Vascular Surgical Service in the venous ulcer clinic at Charing Cross Hospital, Riverside Health Authority, showed that research-based assessment and treatment of chronic venous ulcers substantially improves ulcer healing rates (Blair et al, 1988).

Having already identified that leg ulceration was a community problem it became essential to determine whether research based methods could be implemented within the community with similar results.

Following a successful pilot study in a group practice, the King Edward's Hospital Fund for London awarded its 1988 major grant to a project in Riverside Health Authority, to evaluate the effect of community leg ulcer clinics, implementing a research-based programme of care and supported by the Vascular Surgical Service at Charing Cross.

Research within the Vascular Surgical Service included a programme of assessment and treatment for venous ulceration. This included the development of a high compression bandage system which resulted in a 74 per cent ulcer healing rate at 12 weeks in a vascular clinic (Blair et al, 1988). Simple pinch skin grafting techniques were used to speed the healing of large ulcers (Poskitt et al, 1987), and the provision of elastic hosiery and regular follow-up helped to reduce the rate of ulcer recurrence (Wright et al, 1991).

The innovative aspect of the community project was the development of a close interaction between the Community Unit and a Vascular Surgical Service, providing an integrated service for all patients within the district.

ASSESSING CURRENT PRACTICE

Before implementing a new system of care it was necessary to evaluate the current methods of management and their efficacy. Before the community clinics opened, an audit was carried out by the district nurses working from one health centre. Over 18 weeks 51 patients were treated for a leg ulcer in a total of 865 home visits. At the end of this period the 12 week cumulative healing rate was 22 per cent. The audit also identified that many products were in use and that compression therapy was generally inadequate. This confirmed that many ulcers were failing to heal or taking protracted periods of time.

ESTABLISHING A COMMUNITY LEG ULCER CLINIC

A district-wide network of six community ulcer clinics was developed using existing health centres or clinics to maximise access to the public. Clinics were staffed by the community nurses and supported by specialist nurses from Charing Cross Hospital. Premises were often inadequate to run busy clinics but motivated staff overcame many of these difficulties.

The clinics were developed in partnership with the Community Unit. A period of liaison and consultation with community staff, general practitioners and support services was provided to ensure the most effective service was developed. Posters were strategically placed to heighten public awareness of the new service.

New equipment, such as portable Doppler ultrasound, was purchased by the Community Unit. Only one of the bandages used to apply compression was available on prescription, the remainder being purchased by the Community Unit. This was a very considerable burden at a time of severe financial constraint.

Two district sisters from each health centre acted as co-ordinators for the clinics and were responsible for ordering supplies and running the clinics. They provided continuity for patients as other staff rotated, and had an important teaching role for new staff.

A very close liaison with the specialist nurses was fostered to provide support for the community nurses and to train all staff in the new techniques. Enhanced assessment allowed patients requiring referral to the vascular service to be identified and referred by the specialist nurses. Referral criteria were developed with the vascular surgeons. Patients attending the hospital were seen jointly by the consultant and nurse specialist following full vascular assessment. A programme of care was then negotiated.

TRAINING

The training needs of the project were considerable and occupied a large proportion of specialist nurse time. Problems identified included the sheer number of staff requiring training and the lack of resources and educational structure to meet this need. There was also an ongoing requirement to maintain standards both educationally and clinically to ensure a quality service. A survey of district nurses during the project identified that 98 per cent felt their previous training and experience was inadequate and that a recognised course was required to redress this. The training programme established during the project has culminated in an English National Board course in leg ulcer management.

The Co-ordinator Group

To further ensure integration of acute and community services, a co-ordinator group was established. Co-ordinating sisters met monthly with the specialist nurses at Charing Cross Hospital to participate in training and to discuss any issues arising. This group has been very successful and participates in national study days and the leg ulcer course.

PATIENT ASSESSMENT AND TREATMENT

Assessment

Each patient is holistically assessed to identify any physical, social or psychological factors that may influence progress and need consideration when planning a programme of care. This identifies patients with arterial disease before high compression bandaging is considered. Patients with a reduced pressure index are referred to the hospital for vascular assessment.

Treatment Regime

Simple cleansing: using isotonic normal saline or water.
Skin care: use of bland emollients to enhance skin integrity and prevent dehydration.
Measurement: regular measurement of ulcer area using acetate pen and paper to ensure that ulcer is healing.
Dressings: use of simple, low adherent dressings, as research at Charing Cross Hospital has failed to demonstrate improvement in healing rates by altering the primary dressing (Backhouse et al, 1987).

Four-layer High Compression Bandage Regime

A four-layer bandage system is used to apply 40 mmHg pressure at the ankle graduated to 17 mmHg below the knee. The pressure is maintained for a full week.

Changes in limb circumference are accommodated by a simple ankle circumference measurement which determines the bandages to be used to ensure that the correct pressure is applied to all limbs (table 12.1). Extra padding is used to protect thin, vulnerable limbs and a stronger elasticated bandage is substituted for larger or oedematous limbs.

Table 12.1   Bandage combinations

Ankle circumference	Bandages
Less than 18 cm	two or more Velband; one crepe; one Elset; one Coban
18–25 cm	one Velband; one crepe; one Elset; one Coban
25–30 cm	one Velband; one Plastex 23; one Coban
Greater than 30 cm	one Velband; one Elset; one Plastex 23; one Coban

The bandage combination is determined by the ankle circumference. This should be measured on first assessment and repeated 1 week later when the oedema has reduced.

Pinch Grafting

Large ulcers may benefit from a simple pinch skin grafting technique. This involves removing small pinches of skin from the patient's thigh under local anaesthetic and applying them to a granulating ulcer base. This has the effect of seeding islands of epithelium which grow and unite.

Prevention of Recurrence

When healed, all patients are fitted with a below-knee Class II compression stocking and then seen every 3 months to help reduce the risk of recurrence.

Patient Education

A programme of education begins from the time of assessment. Active patient participation is encouraged and literature is used to reinforce the information given by the nursing staff.

Vascular Assessment

Patients referred to the Vascular Surgical Service include patients with arterial disease, ulcers of other aetiologies or patients failing to progress. Younger patients with venous ulceration or recurrent ulceration are referred to determine whether simple vein surgery may be of benefit. The long term effects of surgery on preventing ulcer recurrence are still unknown. Surgery may be offered as a day case procedure or may involve a 24 hour stay. Hospital referral also allows intervention by other specialities.

TRANSPORT

Providing a cost-effective, efficient community transport service within an inner city area is not without difficulties. Many ulcer patients are too frail or immobile to use public transport to attend a clinic. The Riverside Community clinics required a service that was flexible to their needs and those of the patients. Clinical trials performed within the community clinics raised sufficient funds for the purchase of an adapted ambulance. A driver was recruited, whose compassionate approach with the elderly enhanced this service. It became possible to bring 12 patients, including those with wheelchairs, to each of the six clinics and for many this became the highlight of their week. District Nurses were able to telephone transport requests direct to the driver using an ansaphone system. This system proved extremely cost-effective.

PROBLEMS

The main problems identified in establishing the Riverside service were funding of equipment and bandages, both of which were new financial commitments for the Community Unit. Transport proved more difficult than was first thought and required resourcefulness in looking for alternative methods, which finally resulted in the system outlined above. Community nurses identified increased back strain when 25 patients were seen in one session. This was mainly due to inadequate pump-up couches. Discussion with management resulted in improved facilities and equipment.

PATTERN OF REFERRAL

One of the main aims of the project was to identify all patients with leg ulceration in the district. During a 2 year period 475 patients presented with a leg ulcer to a community clinic. Of these, 46 per cent were referred from the District Nursing service with a further 15 per cent being treated by practice nurses and general practitioners. The two hospital ulcer clinics had been treating 11 per cent of patients. A further 25 per cent of patients self-referred to a community clinic, the majority of whom were unknown to either medical or nursing personnel, and many responded to posters identifying the service. A proportion of these patients were homeless. There is no evidence that the number of patients being referred to the clinics is lessening, with general practitioners fully utilising the service.

Community Patients

The patients treated in the community ulcer clinics were older (74 years median) than those treated in the hospital outpatients (68 years median). Within the district, 11 per cent of patients were either too unwell or immobile to attend a community clinic and were assessed and treated by the community nurses at home. Forty four per cent of all the patients experienced reduced mobility and a third required transport to the clinics.

CAUSES OF ULCERATION

The 475 patients who presented had 550 leg ulcers. Four patients, when first assessed within a community clinic, were thought to have a skin cancer rather than a leg ulcer. These patients were referred to the hospital where biopsy confirmed this, and the appropriate treatment was instigated.

Arterial Disease

Use of Doppler ultrasound identified 56 (10 per cent) patients with significant arterial disease. This was classified as a resting pressure index of 0.5–0.8, and these patients were referred for vascular assessment.

Rheumatoid Arthritis

Eight patients had ulceration related to rheumatoid arthritis.

Diabetes Mellitus

Seven patients presented with foot ulceration. The clinical history and presentation suggested diabetes mellitus to be the causative factor.

In two patients, despite extensive investigation the aetiology could not be determined.

Venous Disease

The remaining 477 ulcers were considered venous in origin and were treated with compression bandaging. The venous ulcers had a median size of 4.2 cm^2 (range 0.1–177 cm^2) with 28 per cent being larger than 10 cm^2. The ulcers were present for a median of 3 months (range 1 week to 63 years) with 27 per cent (150) being present for longer than 1 year.

HEALING RATES

Venous Ulceration

Life table analysis of time to complete healing during the two year period showed that 69 per cent of venous ulcers healed at 12 weeks rising to 83 per cent by 24 weeks.

Mixed Disease

Surprisingly patients with concurrent arterial disease (resting pressure index 0.5–0.8) had a healing rate of 56 per cent at 12 weeks, rising to 75 per cent at 24 weeks. Many of these patients had significant venous disease accompanied by arterial impairment. A regime of reduced compression was used with great care and regular re-assessment using Doppler ultrasound ensured that their arterial status was maintained.

Healing Rate of all Ulcers

The district-wide healing rate for ulcers of all aetiologies during this period was 67 per cent at 12 weeks, rising to 81 per cent at 24 weeks.

RISK FACTORS

A number of risk factors influencing ulcer healing were identified within the Riverside study. These included prolonged ulcer duration, large ulcer size, reduced mobility, poor limb function and treatment at home.

Prolonged ulcer duration and large ulcer size may occur as a consequence of ineffective treatment. Reduced mobility may be an effect rather than a cause of ulceration. Pain around the ulcer site may lead to poor limb mobility and calf function. Patients treated at home healed more slowly than those attending a clinic. However, this group are particularly frail and immobile with other compounding factors influencing their progress. Many of these factors identified can be influenced by providing an effective service where patients are referred at an early stage and receive appropriate treatment.

HEALING RATES OVER TIME

The community clinic healing rates improved over time as the clinics developed. The first group of patients to be treated within the clinics were those already being

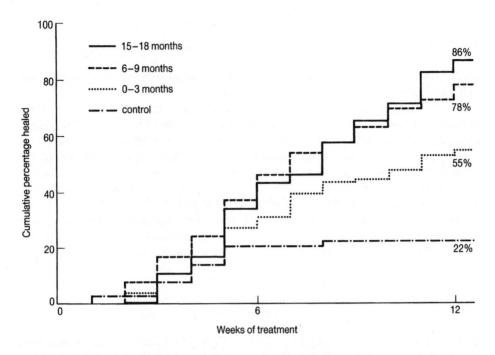

Fig. 12.1 Healing rates of all patients with leg ulceration, by time of referral after start of each clinic and compared with control study (to 12 weeks only).

treated by the district nurses. Although this was a chronic group, the healing rate rose to 55 per cent at 12 weeks within 3 months of the clinics opening. At 6–9 months after opening, the healing rate rose to 78 per cent at 12 weeks and by 15–18 months had risen again to 86 per cent (figure 12.1). This may be a consequence of earlier referral of less chronic ulcers as the service was well known in the area by this time.

PATIENT SATISFACTION

The project sought to assess the degree of patient satisfaction with the service. This was achieved by using a questionnaire which patients completed 12 weeks after commencing treatment and indicated a high level of satisfaction with the service.

QUALITY OF LIFE

Little has been known of the impact of leg ulceration on patients' quality of life. This was assessed using a symptom rating questionnaire, which is a well-validated method of assessing psychiatric morbidity. The questionnaire was completed at the first visit, 12 weeks later and at 48 weeks after referral.

Results from the questionnaire completed at the first visit indicated that patients experienced high levels of anxiety, depression, pain and hostility, and that they experienced significant interference with daily and social activities. By 12 weeks of treatment, when the questionnaire was repeated, there were significant reductions in these levels showing a rapid improvement in the patients' quality of life. Analysis has revealed that this is associated with ulcer healing, with only anxiety reducing in patients whose ulcer failed to heal.

These findings dispel some of the myths concerning leg ulcer patients. Pain was a significant factor experienced by 75 per cent of patients at their first visit and yet it is rarely recognised as a problem relating to venous ulceration.

SUMMARY

The Riverside Community Leg Ulcer Project highlighted the need for an improved service to this group of patients. The project utilised largely existing resources to implement a co-ordinated service, which resulted in improved ulcer healing rates and quality of life for patients.

Provision of an integrated community and acute service ensured patients requiring vascular assessment were promptly referred, with the majority of patients remaining within the community to receive treatment.

The profile of the project raised the status of leg ulceration within the district. It was considered an important developing field where research-based methods had a significant effect on clinical practice. Nursing skills and knowledge were improved and community nurses were able to demonstrate a qualitative aspect of their work.

Changes within the health service demand information on health outcomes. This project allowed management to set realistic targets and to provide evidence to purchasers of a high quality, effective service.

However, this project should not be viewed as a quick answer to a chronic problem; the initiative requires an ongoing investment of time and effort to maintain the level of service. Any new service should be well-supported by an appropriate educational programme that addresses the evolving role of the nurse practitioner in this field.

Leg ulcers are clearly to remain an enormous problem. Demographic changes suggest a 43 per cent increase in those aged over 85 by the year 2000, with the corresponding demand for treatment.

Clinical research indicates that it is realistic to expect 70 per cent of venous ulcers to heal by 12 weeks. We are, however, far from being able to claim that research-based treatments are being used nationally. Detailed clinical research must continue to seek ways of improving healing rates and preventing the depressingly high level of recurrence.

Changes in the NHS should provide incentives to develop new, innovative programmes of care in the community, where there are defined aims and expected outcomes. The availability of compression bandages in the community should enhance these programmes but will bring the very real danger of inappropriate use.

Only through sustained effort can services hope to survive and flourish and patients be relieved of untold misery. It may also be possible to reduce the current bill of £400 million spent on largely ineffective, expensive care.

Acknowledgement

The author thanks the *British Medical Journal* for granting permission to reproduce figure 12.1.

References

Antrobus M (1987) Leg ulcers—establishing the facts. *Geriatric Nursing and Home Care*, **7**(6): 17–18.

Backhouse C M, Blair S D, Walton J and McCollum C N (1987) A controlled trial of occlusive dressings in the healing of chronic venous ulcers. *British Journal of Surgery*, **7**: 626–627.

Bale S (1989) Community nurses awareness of dressing materials. *Care Science and Practice*, **7**(4): 90–92.

Bennett G C J (1992) Undergraduate teaching of chronic wound care. *Lancet*, **339**: 249–250.

Blair S D, Wright D D I, Backhouse C M, Riddle E and McCollum C N (1988) Sustained compression and healing of chronic venous ulcers. *British Medical Journal*, **297**: 1159–1161.

Bosanquet N (1992) Costs of venous ulcers: from maintenance therapy to investment programmes. *Phlebology*, **7** (Suppl 1): 44–46.

Callam M J, Ruckley C V, Harper D R and Dale J J (1985) Chronic ulceration of the leg: extent of the problem and provision of care. *British Medical Journal*, **490**: 1855–1856.

Callam M J, Ruckley C V, Dale J J and Harper D R (1987) Hazards of compression treatment of the leg: an estimate from Scottish Surgeons. *British Medical Journal*, **295**: 1382.

Cameron J (1990) Patch testing for leg ulcer patients. *Nursing Times*, **86**(25): 63–64.

Charles H (1991) Compression healing of ulcers. *Journal of District Nursing*, **10**(3): 4–8, 61–64.

Cockbill S M E (1992) Wound care problems in the community. *Proceedings of the 1st European Conference on Advances in Wound Management*, pp. 3–6. London: Macmillan.

Cornwall J V, Dore C J and Lewis J D (1986) Leg ulcers: epidemiology and aetiology. *British Journal of Surgery*, **73**: 693–696.

Eagle M (1992) Community Clinics. *Nursing Times*, **88**: 46.

Ertl P (1992) A valuable contribution to care. *Professional Nurse*, **7**: 682–688.

Griffey M (1992) Reach for the highest standard. *Professional Nurse*, **8**: 189–192.

Hedges J and Stubbings N (1991) Aspects of treatment in the community. *Prescriber*, **2**(27): 46–55.

Journal of District Nursing (1987) Your data on leg ulcers. *Journal of District Nursing*, **5**(9): 4–6.

Laing W (1992) *Chronic Venous Diseases of the Leg*. London: Office of Health Economics.

Lewis J D and Cornwall J V (1987) The assessment, management and prevention of leg ulcers. *Care of the Elderly*, **1**(2): 82–85.

McIntosh J B (1979) Decision-making on the district. *Nursing Times*, **75**(29): 77–80.

Meyerovitz B R and Nelson R (1964) Measurement of the velocity of blood in lower-limb veins with and without compression. *Surgery*, **56**: 481–486.

Moffatt C J (1992) Compression bandaging—the state of the art. *Journal of Wound Care*, **1**(1): 45–50.

Moffatt C J, Franks P J, Oldroyd M, Bosanquet N, Brown P, Greenhalgh R M and McCollum C N (1992) Community clinics for leg ulcers and impact on healing. *British Medical Journal*, **305**: 1389–1392.

Monk B E and Sarkany I (1982) Outcome of treatment of venous stasis ulcers. *Clinical and Experimental Dermatology*, **72**: 397–400.

Poskitt K R, James A H, Lloyd-Davies E R V, Walton J and McCollum C N (1987) Pinch skin grafting or porcine dermis in venous ulcers: a randomised clinical trial. *British Medical Journal*, **294**: 674–677.

Robinson B (1990) Clinical considerations in the use of compression therapy in the community—a general practitioner's guide. *Care Science and Practice*, **8**(2): 70–71.

Russell G, Bowles A (1992) Developing a community-based leg ulcer clinic. *British Journal of Nursing*, **7**: 337–340.

Ryan T J (1983) *The Management of Leg Ulcers*, p. 64. Oxford: Oxford University Press.

Sigg K (1963) Compression with pressure bandages and elastic stockings for prophylaxis and therapy of venous disorders of the leg. *Fortschrittliche Mediziu*, **15**: 601–606.

Sigel B, Edelstein A L, Felix W R and Memhardt C R (1973) Compression of the deep venous system of the leg during inactive recumbency. *Archives of Surgery*, **106**: 38–43.

Thomas S (1990) Bandages and bandaging: the science behind the art. *Care and Science Practice*, **8**(2): 56–60.

Vydelingum V (1990) Leg ulcer assessment. *Journal of District Nursing*, **8**: 5–10.

Wise G (1986) The social ulcer. *Nursing Times*, **82**(21): 47–49.

Wright D D I, Franks P J, Blair S D, Backhouse C M, Moffatt C J and McCollum C N (1991) Oxerutins in the prevention of recurrence in chronic venous ulceration: a randomized controlled trial. *British Journal of Surgery*, **78**: 1269–1270.

13

Leg Ulcer Research and

Practice: The Way Forward

INTRODUCTION

The preceding chapters have presented us with succinct reviews of the research informing nursing practice in all aspects of leg ulcer management; from the epidemiology of leg ulceration through treatment choice to the organisation of care. When one reads these chapters it becomes clear that despite the commonplace nature of leg ulceration, there is so much that we do not know; about risk factors, about both the primary and secondary prevention of ulceration, about the effectiveness of treatments, and about the efficient delivery of care. We have also seen, in chapter 10, how the uptake of research findings into practice is not always straightforward. This chapter brings together some of the main gaps in our knowledge and suggest the best research strategies for filling them, as well as highlighting some of the areas where practice could be improved with the knowledge we already have.

DEVELOPMENTS IN RESEARCH

Research into the Pathophysiology and Epidemiology of Leg Ulceration

Although there appears to be an association between venous disease and leg ulceration, it is unclear quite how venous incompetence leads to skin breakdown. A number of explanations have been suggested including the fibrin cuff hypothesis (Browse and Burnand, 1982) and the white cell trapping theory (Thomas et al, 1988), but the evidence for each is largely circumstantial. Fundamental research is therefore required to determine the process which leads from venous hypertension to skin ulceration and those factors which inhibit the healing of chronic wounds. Any study which attempts to answer these questions by examining patients with leg ulcers should set inclusion criteria, with a clear definition of what is meant by a leg ulcer. The types of patients which accurately represent the leg ulcer population should be studied, preferably using a random sample of sufficient size. Leg ulcer patients should be compared to age- and sex-matched people without leg ulcers for the parameters of interest.

Well-designed epidemiological studies are needed to determine risk factors for venous disease and venous ulceration so that prevention strategies can be developed. One of the most robust methods for determining causation of disease, the cohort study, is prospective and involves the follow-up of two samples of people; those exposed to the suspected cause of the disease and those not. For example, one may follow up a cohort of individuals from the onset of deep vein thrombosis (DVT) and a group of people who have never experienced a DVT to determine whether the incidence of leg ulceration is greater in the exposed group. As leg ulceration has a relatively low incidence, such a study would need to follow a large sample of people for many years and would therefore be costly. A case-control study on the other hand would involve taking a sample of people who already have leg ulceration and a control group and ascertaining any important differences between them, such as a past history of a DVT. This latter design is by nature retrospective, and therefore much more imprecise, but less costly. Similar studies could also be undertaken to ascertain risk factors for leg ulceration in diabetes and rheumatoid arthritis. Once risk factors have been elucidated, randomised controlled trials of prevention strategies can be undertaken.

Research to Evaluate Leg Ulcer Treatments

Randomized controlled trials (RCTs) are urgently required to answer a number of basic questions about leg ulcer management. The RCT method should be used to explore:

- The optimum level of compression required to heal a venous leg ulcer.
- The most effective bandaging technique to achieve this pressure.
- The consistency and safety of different bandage systems.
- The contribution of different dressings to healing.
- The effectiveness of prophylactic methods such as the wearing of compression hosiery.
- The most effective and efficient means of delivering a leg ulcer service.

It should be stressed that the use of historical controls, in other words comparing the outcomes of a group of patients given a *new* leg ulcer treatment (or other innovation), with the outcomes previously achieved by the old treatment is subject to a myriad of biases and should not be the method of choice. It seems that studies which use a historical control group are much more likely (than an RCT) to conclude that a new treatment is better than the old one (Sacks et al, 1983). The beauty of the randomized controlled trial is that, properly conducted, it should eliminate selection bias (where it is not just the play of chance which determines the intervention which a patient receives in a trial, but some other factor which may influence the outcome as well as the treatment).

Future trials of therapies should involve:

- **Random allocation of the patients to experimental and control groups**. Successful randomisation should be demonstrated in reports of research by presentation of a breakdown of the baseline characteristics of trial participants, e.g. age, sex, duration of ulcer, size of ulcer.

- **The use of sample sizes of sufficient power to demonstrate a clinically important difference, if such a difference exists.** Many leg ulcer studies are of such a small size that any difference between experimental and control treatments would probably not be detected even if one really existed.

- **Clear inclusion and exclusion criteria should be developed** prior to the commencement of any trial. Any evaluation of an innovation in leg ulcer management should observe a well-defined group of patients who have clearly identifiable characteristics. For example, one might expect to get different results if one evaluated the performance of a wound dressing in a group of people with purely venous ulcers compared to a group of people with ulcers of mixed or purely arterial aetiology. The generalisability and clinical relevance of study findings depends on the use and communication of appropriate inclusion and exclusion criteria.

- **Sufficient information should be provided in reports of trials to enable readers to compare the patients studied to those in their own clinical area.** If possible, arterial and venous status should be objectified and reported.

- **The choice of control treatment for comparison within a trial should be appropriate** and should be a reasonable alternative to the product under study. Some trials have been confounded by the use of a control treatment which may actively inhibit healing, so making the new product look more effective.

- **The *only* difference between the patients in the control and the treatment group should be the product or intervention in question.** For example, it is important to standardise such variables as compression bandaging in a trial which compares the effect of two dressings on venous ulcer healing.

- **Trials should be of sufficient duration to demonstrate complete healing rates.** The complete healing of an ulcer is a clear endpoint, and the only endpoint of interest to clinicians and patients. Many studies are only of 6 or 8 weeks duration, in which time few ulcers will have completely healed. Healing *rates* are notoriously difficult to measure accurately, and it is far easier and more meaningful to compare the numbers of patients whose ulcers have completely healed at a certain time, across the two or more intervention groups. Good examples of this type of study have been done by Blair et al (1988) and Callam et al (1992).

- **All clinically relevant outcomes should be reported in the results of a trial, including complete healing rates and any adverse effects occurring in either treatment or control group.** Outcome measures such as the degree of granulation and/or cleansing at time points in advance of healing are not sufficient on their own to demonstrate effectiveness. It is important to know whether there is any effect on total healing time even where products are only used for a phase of the treatment period.

- **All patients who have participated in a clinical trial should be accounted for.** It should be clear how many people entered and completed the trial; any discrepancy between these figures (due to the withdrawal or death of patients) should be accounted for. It should be clear how many people withdrew from each treatment group.

● It is useful if **additional data such as patient comfort and satisfaction, frequency of dressing or bandage changes and nursing time required to apply the treatments are collected and reported.**

● **The issue of contact sensitivity requires further study**, particularly in relation to the clinical history of contact sensitivity including how it may change over time, how it may best be detected by the community nurse and how its occurrence may be minimised. The possibility of new dressings with little or no tendency to induce an allergic response should be explored.

DEVELOPMENTS IN PRACTICE

● **The primary health care team requires education concerning the management of patients with leg ulcers.** Both general practitioners and nurses need to know how to assess leg ulcer patients; paying particular attention to the evaluation of arterial circulation and screening for diabetes and rheumatoid arthritis.

● **An assessment of a patient's experience of pain should be part of every assessment and appropriate advice regarding analgesia should be given or analgesia prescribed if necessary.**

● **Clear criteria should be developed and agreed locally to direct the referral of patients who may require a specialist vascular, dermatological or other opinion.** A successful leg ulcer service is dependent on good links between the hospital and community.

● **The relatively good mobility of many leg ulcer patients** suggests that delivery of leg ulcer care from a clinic base may be a more efficient use of nurse-time, and would also promote exercise and social contact between leg ulcer patients.

● **The ingredients of leg ulcer preparations should be clearly listed on packaging and patients known to be allergic to a component of treatment should be given clear, written information about what products to avoid in the future.** Awareness of contact sensitivity as a clinical problem should be raised with the primary health care team and patients referred to dermatology departments for patch testing.

● **Patients should be followed-up after ulcer healing, in order to promote compliance with compression hosiery and anticipate imminent skin breakdown.**

References

Blair S D, Wright D D, Backhouse C M, Riddle E and McCollum C N (1988) Sustained compression and healing of chronic venous ulcers. *British Medical Journal*, **297**: 1159–1161.
Browse N L and Burnand K G (1982) The cause of venous ulceration. *Lancet*, **ii**: 243–245.
Callam M J, Harper D R, Dale J J, Brown D, Gibson B, Prescott R J and Ruckley C V (1992) Lothian and Forth Valley Leg Ulcer Healing Trial Part 2: knitted viscose dressing

versus a hydrocellular dressing in the treatment of chronic leg ulceration. *Phlebology*, **7**: 142–145.

Sacks H S, Chalmers T C and Smith H (1983) Sensitivity and specificity of clinical trials: randomized versus historical controls. *Archives of Internal Medicine*, **143**: 753–755.

Thomas P R, Nash G B and Dormandy J A (1988) White cell accumulation in dependent legs of patients with venous hypertension: a possible mechanism for trophic changes in the skin. *British Medical Journal*, **296**: 1693–1695.

Index

Page numbers in **bold type** refer to figures; those in *italics* refer to tables.

accidents, as cause of traumatic ulcers 13
adhesive bandages 70
adhesives, as allergens 107, *107*
advice to patients, research studies 118–19
age, and prevalence of ulcers *20, 21*
alginate dressings 54–5
allergens *104*, 105–7, *107*
amerchol, as allergen 105, *107*
anaesthetics, local, as allergens 107
ankle: brachial pressure index (ABPI) 31–2
ankle joint mobility 30
ankle systolic pressure 32
antibiotics, topical
    as allergens 105–6, *107*
    in dressings 117
antiseptics, for wound cleansing 42, 44, 116
anxiety 131
appearance, of ulcers 33–4
arterial (ischaemic) ulcers 11, **14**
    appearance of 33
    factors associated with *31*
arteries 1
arterioles 1
assessment, *see* nursing assessment; patient
    assessment
assessment forms **28–9**
'atrophie blanche' 31

balsam of Peru, as allergen 106, *107*
bandages
    adhesive/cohesive 70
    compression bandages 69
    conformability of 66
    conforming stretch 68
    elasticity of 66
    extensibility of 66
    light support 68–9
    and modulus 66

and power 66
properties of 66
support by 66
tubular 70
washing, effect of 79
see also extensible bandages; paste ban-
    dages; stretch bandages
bandaging
    aim of 75–7
    four-layer system, in Riverside project
        140–1
    research studies 117–18
    terms and definitions 66
    see also pressure, sub-bandage
bandaging techniques
    bandage extension 83–4
    criss-cross method 82–3
    figure of eight 82–3
    overlap 84
    with paste bandages 83
    positioning of patient 81
    with problem legs 85–6
    problems with 84
    with short-stretch bandages 83
    simple spiral 81–2
    spica 82–3
batteries (allergen groups) 104
bead dressings
    cadexomer iodine 50, *52*
    dextranomer 49–50, *51*
benzocaine, as allergen 107
biocides, as allergens 106, *107*
Biofilm, trials of 48
blood flow
    in arteries 1
    in capillaries 2
    and hydrostatic pressure 64
    in veins and venules 2, 3–6

blood pressure, in nursing assessment 30
blood samples 30
brachial systolic pressure 32
burns, as cause of traumatic ulcers 13

cadexomer iodine 50, *52*
calf muscle pump 3–5, **6**, 63
capillaries 2
capillary filling, assessment of 31
capillary permeability 10
carba mix, as allergen 106, *107*
care, *see* treatment
causes of ulceration, in Riverside project 143
cetyl alcohol, *see* cetylstearyl alcohol
cetylstearyl alcohol, as allergen 106, *107*
chlorhexidine, as allergen 106
chloroxylenol, as allergen 106, *107*
circulation, venous 3–6
cleansers, *see* wound cleansers
cleansing, *see* wound cleansing
clinics
    establishment of 139
    and patient mobility 152
cohesive bandages 70
colophony, as allergen 107, *107*
Comfeel, trials of 47–8, 48–9
compliance
    and compression hosiery 96
    and re-ulceration 90
    research findings 120–1
compression
    definition 66
    graduated external 64–5
    as important treatment method 137
    misuse, dangers of 72, 137
    relative performances of different bandages 71–2
    role of 63–5
compression bandages 69
compression bandaging, research studies 117–18
compression hosiery
    amount of pressure 91–2
    British Standard for 65
    classes of 91, *92*
    contra-indications 97
    fitting 94, **95**
    function of 91
    graduated compression 92
    after healing of ulcer 111
    history 91
    lifespan of 96–7
    need for follow-up 96
    and patient compliance 96
    testing methods 92–3
    types of 93–4
    washing 96–7
conformability, of bandages 66
constraints, on nursing practice 120
contact dermatitis 103
    allergic 103, *see also* allergens; patch testing
    irritant 103, 109
    management of 109
contact sensitivity 101, *102*
    prevention of 110
    and product labelling 152
    studies of 108
    see also allergens
criss-cross bandaging 82–3

debridement
    chemical 42, 44
    enzymic 44–5
    see also wound cleansing
Debrisan 49–50, *51*
deep vein thrombosis (DVT), as predisposing factor 5, 23–4
deep veins 4
demography, and risk of ulcers 22–3
depression 125–6, 131
dermatitis, *see* contact dermatitis
dextranomer 49–50, *51*
diabetic ulcers 13
    appearance of 33
diagnosis, research studies 113–14
diet 30
Doppler ultrasound 31–2
    prevention of wrong treatment 136
dorsalis pedis pulse (DP) 31
dressings
    alginate 54–5
    bead dressings 49–50, *51–2*
    danger of pressure necrosis 87
    paste bandages 50, 53–5, 83
    research studies 117
    in Riverside project 140
    trials of *43*
    see also bandages; hydrocolloid dressings; Unna boots

Duoderm, *see* Granuflex
DVT, *see* deep vein thrombosis
dyes, as allergens 107

eczema 102
  acute, management of 109–10
  endogenous 102, *see also* venous stasis
    eczema
  exogenous 102, *see also* contact dermatitis
education, for nurses 121, 122
  need for 152
  in Riverside project 142
elasticity, of bandages 66
endogenous eczema 102, *see also* venous
  stasis eczema
energy loss 130–1
enzymic debridement 44–5
epidemiology, need for research into 149–50
ester gum resin, as allergen 107, *107*
eucerin, as allergen 105, *107*
European Standard Battery *104*
exogenous eczema 102, *see also* contact dermatitis
extensibility, of bandages 66
extensible bandages
  classification 67–9
  compression bandages, types of 69
  development of 65–6
  light support 68–9
  lightweight conforming stretch bandages
    68

fibrin cuffs 10–11, **12**
fibrinogen 10
figure of eight bandaging 82–3
follow-up, need for 152
foot pulses 31–2
foot pump 5
fragrance mix, as allergen 106, *107*
framycetin, as allergen 105, *107*

gaiter area 32, **33**
gentamicin, as allergen 105, *107*
grafts, *see* skin grafting
Granuflex (Duoderm)
  and permeability 45
  trials of 46–7, 48–9

haemolytic ulcers 13
healing

patients after 111
  rates of, in Riverside project 144, 144–5
  see also wound healing
health services, involvement of 21–2
hosiery, *see* compression hosiery
hydrocolloid dressings
  choice of 48–9
  and permeability 45
  studies of 46–9
hydrogen peroxide, as wound cleanser 116
hypochlorites, and wound cleansing 42

incidence 17
International Contact Dermatitis Research
  Group (ICDRG), guidelines 104
Iodosorb 50, *52*
ischaemic disease 30–1
ischaemic ulcers, *see* arterial ulcers

lanolin, as allergen 105, *107*
Laplace equation 66–7
leg ulcers
  causes of 1
  definition 9
  factors associated with *2*
  formation of **12**
  more common on left leg 5–6
  see also ulcers
legs
  bandaging techniques 85–6
  vascular system 1–7
life style, effect on 128
light support bandage 68–9
lipodermatosclerosis 10, 102
living conditions, patient's 27, 30
local anaesthetics, as allergens 107
lock out 66, 68
lymphatics 2
lymphoedema 2

malignant ulcers 13
  appearance of 34
medical history, and risk of ulcers 23, 30
mercapto, as allergen 106, *107*
microorganisms, and wound healing 39–40
mixed aetiology ulcers, factors associated
  with *31*
mobility 129
  of ankle joint 30
modulus, and bandage length 66

moisture, and wound healing 38–9
muscle pumps, *see* calf muscle pump; foot
    pump

necrosis, *see* pressure necrosis
neomycin, as allergen 105–6, *107*
noncompliance, *see* compliance
nurses
    and choice of treatment 116
    constraints on practice 120
    sources of information 121
    and year of qualification 114–15, 121
nursing assessment
    accurate diagnosis essential 27
    assessment forms **28–9**
    elements of 27, 30–4
    surveys of 114–16
    see also patient assessment
nursing practice
    constraints on 120
    development of 122, 132–3, 152

occupation, patient's 27
oedema 32, *see also* lymphoedema
oxygen, and wound healing 39

pain 33, 130, *131*
    need for assessment and advice 152
    research studies 118–19
parabens, as allergen 106, *107*
paste bandages 50, 53–5, 83
patch testing 104–5
    in clinical practice 108–9
    negative results 105
pathophysiology, need for research into
    149–50
patient assessment
    in Riverside project 140, 141–2
    see also nursing assessment
patient satisfaction, in Riverside project 145
patients' perceptions, research study
    anxiety and depression 131
    awareness of ulcer 128
    current research 126
    energy loss 130–1
    health measures 130–1
    knowledge of leg ulcers 127–8
    life style, effect on 128
    mobility 129
    pain 130, *131*

participants in 127
patients' feelings 128
previous research 125–6
problems experienced *131*
recommendations 132–3
sleep 130
social contact 129
ulcer management 132
perforators 4
perfumes, as allergens 106, *107*
peripheral arterial disease 11
phenosept, as allergen 106, *107*
p-phenylenediamine (PPD), as allergen 107
pinch grafting 56, 141
posterior tibial pulse (PTP) 31
posture
    and blood flow 64
    effect on bandage pressure 79, **80**
    and venous blood pressure 2
power, and bandage length 66
preservatives, as allergens 106, *107*
pressure, sub-bandage
    clinical assessment 76
    decrease with time 79
    factors influencing 66–7
    formula for 66–7
    measurement of 76–8
    variation with posture 79, **80**
pressure gradient 77–8
pressure monitors 78
pressure necrosis
    and dressings 87
    minimising 86
    and support stockings 97
    vulnerable areas 87
prevalence
    and age 20, *21*
    from case ascertainment 20–1
    definition 17
    from opportunistic surveys 19–20
    using questionnaires 18–19
    from sample of at-risk population 18
pulse, *see* foot pulses
pumps, *see* calf muscle pump; foot pump

quality of life, and Riverside project 145
questionnaire surveys, for estimation of
    prevalence 18–19
quinoline mix, as allergen 106, *107*

re-ulceration
  factors influencing 90
  follow-up trials 90, 119
  prevention of 89
  recurrence rates 89–90
  referral as method of prevention 119
  risk groups 90
recurrence, see re-ulceration
referrals
  low number of 119
  need for criteria 122, 152
  in Riverside project 142
research
  basis for practice 35
  further need for 149–52
  see also under individual subjects
resting pressure index (RPI), see ankle:
  brachial pressure index
rheumatoid arthritis 13, 30
rheumatoid ulcers 13, 30
  appearance of 34
risk factors
  deep vein thrombosis (DVT) 23–4
  demographic 22–3
  and medical history 23
  in Riverside project 144
Riverside community project
  background 138
  causes of ulceration 143
  community patients 143
  establishment of clinics 139
  healing rates 144, 144–5
  patient assessment and treatment 140–2
  patient satisfaction 145
  preliminary audit 139
  problems 142
  quality of life 146
  referral 142
  risk factors 144
  training 139–40
  transport 142
rubber mixes, as allergens 106, 107

saline, as wound cleanser 116
sensitivity, see contact sensitivity
sensitizers, see allergens
short-stretch bandages 68–9, 83
sickle cell anaemia, as cause of haemolytic
  ulcers 13
simple spiral bandaging 81–2

site of ulcer 32
skin grafting 55–6, 141
sleep 130
smoking 11, 30
social contact 129
spica bandaging 82–3
stearyl alcohol, see cetylstearyl alcohol
stockings, see compression hosiery
streptokinase-streptodornase, clinical trials
  44–5
stretch bandages
  lightweight conforming 68
  short (minimal) 68–9, 83
sub-bandage pressure, see pressure, sub-
  bandage
superficial veins 4, **5**
support, by bandages 66
support stockings, see compression hosiery

thiuram mix, as allergen 106, *107*
topical antibiotics
  as allergens 105–6, *107*
  in dressings 117
training, see education
transport, and Riverside project 142
traumatic ulcers 13
treatment
  cost of 135–6
  generally ineffective 137
  need for research into 150–2
  in Riverside project 140
  studies of 137–8
  use of inappropriate products 136–7
trypsin, clinical trials 44–5
tubular bandages 70

ulcers
  arterial, see arterial ulcers
  diabetic 13, 33
  haemolytic 13
  ischaemic, see arterial ulcers
  malignant 13, 34
  of mixed aetiology, factors associated
    with *31*
  rheumatoid 13, 30
  traumatic 13
  varicose 10
  venous, see venous ulcers
  see also leg ulcers
ultrasound, see Doppler ultrasound

Unna boots 50, 54
    trials of 46–7
urinalysis 30

valves, venous 2, **4**, **7**, **11**
varicose ulcers 10
varicose veins **11**, 30
vascular disease, cause of leg ulcers 1
vehicles, as allergens 106, *107*
veins, 2, **3**, **7**
    anatomy differences 5–6
    circulation in 3–6
    communicating (perforators) 4
    deep 4
    superficial 4, **5**
    valves in 2, **4**, **7**
    varicose **11**, 30
venous disease, main cause of leg ulcers 1, *9*
venous reflux 4
venous sinus 2, **4**
venous stasis (varicose) eczema 102–3
    management of 110
venous ulcers 10–11
    appearance of 33
    factors associated with *31*
venules 2

walking, as aid to circulation 5, 63
weight, patient's 30
wool alcohols, as allergens 105, *107*
wound care
    research studies 36–7
    as a speciality 137–8
wound cleansers, chemical 42
wound cleansing
    current opinion 44
    enzymic debridement 44–5
    research studies 116
    in Riverside project 140
    use of antiseptics 42, 44, 116
wound healing
    barriers to 41
    and devitalised tissue 40–1
    and microorganisms 39–40
    and moisture 38–9
    and oxygen 39
    the process 37–8
    see also healing
wound management
    objectives of 41–2
    see also bandaging; dressings; wound
        cleansing